M000222825

THIS BOOK COULD SAVE YOUR LIFE.

THIS BOOK COULD SAVE YOUR LIFE.

Breaking the silence around the mental health emergency

BEN WEST

HarperCollins*Publishers*

HarperCollins*Publishers*
1 London Bridge Street
London SE1 9GF

www.harpercollins.co.uk

HarperCollinsPublishers
1st Floor, Watermarque Building, Ringsend Road
Dublin 4, Ireland

First published by HarperCollins*Publishers* 2022

10 9 8 7 6 5 4 3 2 1

A catalogue record of this book is available from the British Library

ISBN 978-0-00-850314-7

Printed and bound in the UK using 100% renewable electricity at CPI Group (UK) Ltd

MIX
Paper from
responsible sources
FSC™ C007454

This book is produced from independently certified FSC™ paper to ensure responsible
forest management.

For more information visit: www.harpercollins.co.uk/green

To my brother, Sam. I miss you.
I still haven't stopped and I'm still trying.

CONTENTS

A note from Ben   1

Introduction   5

1   A normal family   21
2   21/01/2018   53
3   WTF just happened?   85
4   Walk to Talk   119
5   'Hi Boris, can I have a word?'   151
6   Burnout   193
7   All in the name of academic excellence   221
8   A letter from the future   255

Final thoughts   277
Useful websites/resources/further reading   281
References   285
Acknowledgements   293

A NOTE FROM BEN

Thank you so much for picking up this book. Any friend of mine will tell you that the fact I've even written one is more than a little surprising – to say I was the least likely one of us to become an author is an understatement. At primary school I was told by my teacher not to bother sitting my English exams because it would be 'demoralising' for me. (Turns out it was more demoralising to be told it'd be demoralising. Go figure.) Before you sigh and put it back on the shelf though, I've got a brilliant editor who's been fab and has assured me that despite my lack of qualifications it does actually make sense. Phew. But previous to this, I had always struggled with words – finding the right ones and getting them on paper in a way that made sense. Then, in January 2018, something happened that suddenly forced me to find the words, come what may: the suicide of my younger brother, Sam.

Sam took his own life, aged 15, five months after being diagnosed with clinical depression. This book details my personal journey in dealing with the shock, grief and realisation that Sam's death, like many other deaths caused by mental illness, could possibly have been avoided. Had Sam received the support he needed and if we all talked about mental health in a different way, perhaps there would be no need for this book. Damn, how I wish that were the case.

Before we dive fully into that though, it's time for a proper introduction.

Hello. My name is Ben West. I'm 22 years old. You might know me from Instagram, where I split my time between breaking down stigmas, campaigning for change and responding to many of my followers' horrifically detailed confessions while dressed in a priest outfit. Or perhaps you recognise me from the time I closed the 2019 ITV election debate by asking the prime minister, Boris Johnson, and the leader of the opposition at the time, Jeremy Corbyn, the question that was on everyone's lips: 'What would you buy each other for Christmas?' Alternatively, maybe you haven't the faintest idea who I am, but were drawn to the title of this book because mental health is something you, or someone you know, is struggling with. Whatever brought you here – welcome! I really appreciate you being interested in my story and I hope you find it useful.

People often say to me, 'Wow, you've been so unlucky', which simply isn't true. I've actually been nothing but lucky. I'm lucky because on 21 January 2018 two very different situations were playing out in my house: I was lying on my bed listening to music and my brother was lying on his floor taking his own life. I'm lucky because I've seen how easy it would've been for me to have been in his place. I'm lucky that I haven't had to face the darkness that comes with depression and mental illness. I'm lucky that I don't have to gamble my life on an under-resourced and failing NHS support system. I'm lucky that my parents' financial situation doesn't determine whether I live or die. And I'm lucky that my postcode doesn't change the quality of care I have access to.

Sam's death has forced me to recognise and acknowledge this luck – and I'm livid about it. It is what drove me to become a mental health campaigner and to write this book, because the suggestion that any of this is down to luck is bullshit. Nothing will ever change if we sit down and stay quiet. We *must* stand up and speak out. We must find the words, regardless of the challenges or the barriers.

The words in this book are a plea for change. I want to help change how helpless you feel if you're suffering right now, or if you know someone who is; I want to change how we speak about mental health and suicide; and I want to change governmental policy. It's not okay any more for people to wander about, blissfully unaware that this other deadly pandemic is going on. It *is* going on, and it's about time we fucking did something about it.

I'll consider this book to have done its job if it makes you feel sad but supported, seen and less alone, inspired and motivated, overwhelmed but aware. We all have a responsibility to speak up when we see suffering and injustice and when we're in a position to help others. We must find the words, and these are mine.

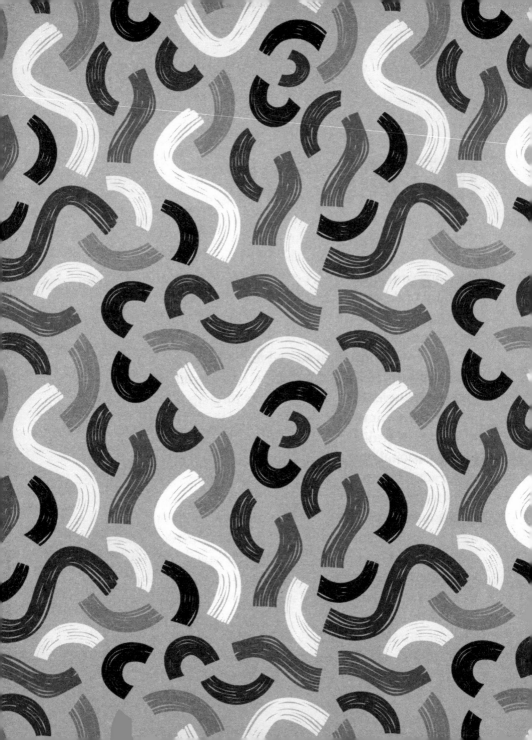

INTRODUCTION

How are you? Fine? That's great. How about happy, though? Would you describe yourself as happy? Content? Pretty zen? Ticking along? Or are you, if you're being really honest, none of those things?

I believe the most important commodity in life is happiness. The ability to feel joy. Happiness means different things to different people. Being generally 'happy' doesn't mean you're punching the air with euphoria every second of every day (that would be unrealistic and highly inconvenient), but it means that occasionally you do feel that way. And sure, you also feel awful sometimes – even *really* awful – but it's temporary. You know that emotions pass and that the sadness, angst or general meh you feel is a necessary part of processing what's going on in your life. When you're down, you know that tomorrow, or the week or month after that, you'll probably feel a bit better. Hell, when that happens you may even punch the air. Why not?

However, a lot of people don't ever feel better. Their emotions *don't* pass. They're stuck in the 'I feel like shit' lane and can't get out. To lose a sense of happiness entirely is to lose everything and I feel an immense amount of empathy towards those many, many people who wake up every single day unhappy.

On which cheerful note: welcome to my book! Come on in – there are actually laughs inside, I promise!

THIS BOOK COULD SAVE YOUR LIFE: WHAT'S IT ALL ABOUT?

I believe the UK, and much of the world, is in the grips of a mental health emergency, and that, no matter how you dress up the facts and figures, no one can deny that the rate of mental illness is deeply, deeply concerning. This book is about what I've discovered during the past four years – after throwing myself into the deep end of all things mental health, both personally and publicly. Here's a taster of what I've learned.

A quarter of all adults will experience some form of mental illness every year in the UK,[1] while three children in an average UK classroom will have a diagnosable mental health issue.[2, 3] Those numbers contribute to the 834,000,000 people (yes, you read that right) who are estimated to be suffering from a mental health disorder around the world.[4]

It's easy to become numb to statistics – especially when the figures are so huge. Be honest, I bet your eyes glazed over reading that last bit and you started thinking, 'Hmm ... what shall I make for dinner tonight?' So, let me put it another way: every single one of those numbers represents an actual person, and if that person is lucky enough to have a caring community of people around them, that community will be directly affected too.

When you start to think about how many people are touched by mental health issues – such as depression, anxiety, eating disorders, body dysmorphia, PTSD, OCD, to name just a few – you quickly realise that it would be a very rare person indeed who isn't affected at all. If you're not suffering yourself, you most likely know someone who is. And, with Covid-19 having stomped all over our lives, the only word I can use to describe how I feel, as someone who works within the mental health space, is fear. I am genuinely terrified about how rapidly these numbers might rack up over the coming years.

So our collective mental health is shot to shit. But, it's okay because there are systems in place to help us all out. Right? RIGHT?

Well, let's talk about that.

Who and what has been tasked with the mammoth job of keeping our minds vaguely functioning? The UK's mental health service. Before I say anything else on this, I want to clarify that the majority of the people I've come into contact with who work within the mental health service are inspirational individuals performing an incredibly difficult job to the very best of their ability under ridiculous amounts of pressure. I want to shout that as loudly as possible, so imagine me standing on a stage screaming into a megaphone, 'THEY ARE

HEROES!', please. And remember that image as I continue, because within this book I'll reveal just what a shitshow the state of those services are and just what those people are having to deal with.

What is at fault is the fact that demand for services is huge and available resources are simply not adequate. Between April 2019 and March 2020 (so pre-lockdown), 538,564 children and young people were referred to the Child and Adolescent Mental Health Service (CAMHS). Of those referrals, 70 per cent (376,995) weren't seen at all within three months. Twenty-seven per cent had their referrals closed (which is also known as the 'rejection rate' . . . yeah . . .), while 36 per cent were either contacted once during that period or weren't contacted at all.[5] Put another way: young people will wait an average of 53 days to receive NHS care from a specialist for their mental illness – nearly double the government's four-week target.[6]

At the time of writing, the figures for April 2020–March 2021 aren't available, so we don't yet know what impact repeated lock-downs and pandemic restrictions will have had on the demand for this service. I fear though that it's been the perfect storm. Things were already dire pre-Covid – it doesn't take a crystal-ball-bothering psychic to predict that they won't have got any better during the maddest and most tempestuous few years in living memory. Already, post-lockdown, we are seeing urgent mental health referrals hit the highest levels ever recorded.[7]

A health service is there to treat someone when they need it, but unfortunately, for so many people, help isn't available, or when it is, it simply isn't good enough.

FOR TOO LONG WE HAVE TALKED AND TALKED AND *TALKED* ABOUT HOW IMPORTANT DEALING WITH MENTAL ILLNESS AND PREVENTING SUICIDE IS, AND FOR FAR TOO LONG THAT CONVERSATION HAS ENDED WITH A FULL STOP.

THIS IS PERSONAL

I was forced to discover all of this following my brother's suicide in January 2018 after a diagnosis of clinical depression. When Sam died, I didn't know what mental illness was, I didn't know what depression was, and, had you asked my view on 'the mental health crisis', I'd have blankly shrugged and asked what you meant. Over the past few years, my understanding of both the bigger and smaller pictures (as regards my own mental health) has grown exponentially. This book is both a glimpse into my personal experience of tackling the excruciating pain that came with the grief and trauma of Sam's death – and a call for change.

For too long we have talked and talked and *talked* about how important dealing with mental illness and preventing suicide is, and for far too long that conversation has ended with a full stop. We need change, we need it now, and my hope is that this book will be a catalyst for exactly that. When Sam died it became my priority to try to prevent another individual enduring what Sam did, and another family going through what ours did. Campaigners like myself, charities, advocates, experts and mental health workers are all trying their hardest, but in the four years following Sam's death, around 20,000 other families in England and Wales have gone through the same thing we experienced.[8, 9, 10]

I won't lie to you: that fact sometimes makes me want to jack it all in, grab a beer and go live in a cave, but actually, while that number grows, so does my passion and my determination to fight.

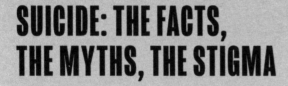

SUICIDE: THE FACTS, THE MYTHS, THE STIGMA

What is suicide? Suicide is when people harm themselves with the intention of ending their own life, and they die as a result, while a 'suicide attempt' is when someone harms themselves with the intention of ending their life, and they do not die.[11]

WHY MIGHT SOMEONE TAKE THEIR OWN LIFE?

There are many reasons a person may choose to end their life. Some of the most common are:

* ✳ Severe depression and/or mental illness.
* ✳ Substance-abuse-influenced impulsivity.
* ✳ Traumatic stress (such as abuse or being the victim of a violent crime).
* ✳ Loss or fear of loss (such as academic failure, the end of a relationship, loss of a job).
* ✳ Hopelessness (a symptom of depression, but also a stand-alone response to a one-off situation that a person cannot see a way out of).

»

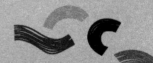

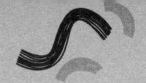

* Chronic pain or illness.
* Feeling a burden to others.
* A cry for help (e.g. not necessarily wanting to die, but not wanting to live the life they have).

THE NUMBERS

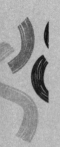

In 2019, there were 5,691 recorded suicides in the UK[12] and approximately 700,000 suicides worldwide.[13] It is estimated that each year in England and Wales at least 140,000 people are hospitalised after attempting suicide.[14] (According to WHO, a prior suicide attempt is the single most important risk factor for suicide in the general population.[15])

THE STIGMA

Stigmas surrounding suicide are historical, societal and cultural. Attempting suicide was an actual *crime* in the UK until 1961. Imagine that – being arrested for a suicide attempt, which is often the symptom of an illness. That's like the police breaking into a cancer hospice and having to explain to grieving relatives that they'll need to take statements because, 'I'm sorry, but dying from an illness is now fucking illegal.'

That law around suicide still has an impact today, fuelling prejudice and misinformation. Don't believe me? How many times have you heard the phrase 'committed suicide'? Probably too many times to count. It's related to the language of crime: commit murder,

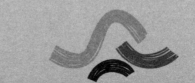

commit suicide. This association – no matter how unintended nowadays – helps to maintain the belief that suicide is in some way 'wrong', a moral failure or a weakness of character, which exacerbates the taboo around the subject. It's only recently, now people are becoming more sensitive to the language around mental health, that this damaging phrase is losing its prevalence. (Better phrases to use include 'died by suicide', 'took their own life', or simply 'killed him/her/themself'.)

Then there's the religious angle. Within some religions, suicide is considered a sin as only God has the right to take life. People who kill themselves, therefore, are not (or were not) allowed to be buried in consecrated ground.

The societal and cultural complexities surrounding the subject are deep and getting into them is not what this book is about. But, suffice to say that connecting all these stigmas is the idea that the person who has died has done something wrong, ergo the subject is uncomfortable or taboo. This causes a reluctance to talk about it, to address it, and to understand it.

THE FACTS

The truth is, suicide is not a crime, it's a tragedy; it's not a choice, it's a symptom. There is a misconception that to be suicidal, or to attempt suicide, is to be weak or attention seeking, but I've spoken to many people who have either contemplated taking their own lives or who have tried, and they are the strongest, most inspiring people I've ever met.

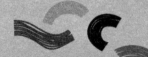

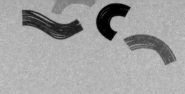

There is nothing weak about waking up every day to a brain that tells you that those you love would be better off if you were dead or that things are hopeless. To be able to endure that level of despair for any amount of time takes immeasurable courage. But one can only be so strong for so long, and losing that fight is not weak – it is inevitable without the right help.

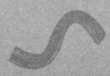

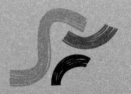

PRETTY VS UGLY

There are two conversations about mental health: the pretty one and the ugly one.

The pretty conversation: 'It's important to talk about mental health! Now, what's for lunch?'

Advocating that everyone should talk more about mental health is a nice-looking soundbite that brands, companies and politicians tweet, slap on billboards and base Instagram campaigns around. And, while yes, OF COURSE it's important that people are encouraged to talk about mental health – my God, that's a key part of this entire book – we have to go further than that. How and where should people talk about it? To whom? And what should they do if they can't?

Those kinds of we're-all-in-it-together comments, reeled off with little substance to back them up, trivialise an incredibly complex issue. Oh, everyone should just chat more? Great. Job done. Off we go. Instead, we *must* learn to talk about the stuff that doesn't look good on billboards, that would get content warnings on Twitter, and that would create a *very* uncomfortable silence if a politician really got into it while opening the local village fete.

The ugly conversation: 'People are talking, they are reaching out for support, and they're not getting it. They're still dying.'

The ugly conversation is the reality of mental illness: the reality of having to deal with the fact that a loved one's suicide may have been preventable had they received timely and adequate support. And the reality that, had we all been better prepared to have ugly conversations, maybe I wouldn't have needed to write this book.

A week after Sam died my family were contacted by the NHS mental health service telling us that there was now a counselling session available for him. I mean, can you imagine? It was like falling down a 100-foot well and finding a penny. Cheers, Universe. And Sam had been *actively* seeking support and engaging with all the appropriate services. What was offered was too little, far too late.

Unfortunately, for a lot of people the story isn't much better even if they *do* get into the service in time. Mental health workers are under extraordinary pressure; the system is bursting at the seams. The disparity between what I hear from politicians and what the people on the front line within mental health units tell me is striking. CAMHS has previously been described by ministers as 'robust and well-resourced'. How do they justify having that kind of 'pretty conversation' with someone who's been waiting for help for over a year?

To me, an apt visual summary of the current conversations surrounding mental health is the meme of a dog drinking a cup of tea in a room that's on fire and saying, 'This is fine.'

REAL-LIFE EXAMPLES OF NECESSARY UGLY CONVERSATIONS

An A&E nurse once told me that he treated a woman who'd had a panic attack lasting several days. She was so anxious she couldn't eat without vomiting and had soiled herself. When the mental health team was contacted, they said they wouldn't see her because she wasn't suicidal and deemed at high enough risk for care. She was discharged.

Another person was refused NHS help for an eating disorder because they weren't underweight enough. The young person and her parents agreed that they would let the eating disorder get worse – and risk a heart attack – so they could be accepted into the programme.

A mother of a primary school girl told me her daughter tried to take her own life in the playground at school after her best friend died. The school's response was to suspend her for scaring the other children.

The University of Lancaster's response to one of their students self-harming during lockdown was to transfer him to empty student accommodation. He was forced to isolate during lockdown entirely alone. He attempted suicide.[16]

While these stories are shocking, they are real and are happening every day – and if we're serious about trying to solve the mental health crisis, we need to do more to listen and to try to understand them. We also need to call for systemic change. That's why within this book you'll find tips on how to start these ugly conversations, how to listen to them and how to respond.

WHY READ THIS BOOK

Since I was 17, I've thrown myself into learning everything I can about mental health. Not just about the systems that are – or aren't – in place to help people, but about my own emotions and ways of processing the things that happen to me.

I've always said that I think it would be very beneficial if everyone could have been through what I've been through, without having to lose a loved one. I wish everyone could have met the people I've met, seen what I've seen, done what I've done, and felt what I've felt. It's those experiences that have built me up to be the campaigner and person I am today.

It's a rollercoaster ride – one of agony, anger, elation and laughter – and I'm inviting you to join me on it. Strap in because I want this book to make you cry with me and laugh with (and sometimes at) me. I want it to make you feel angry, hopeful and inspired. But, most of all, I want you to come away knowing that you can help. That there are things you can do to help yourself, your friends, your family, and people you've never even met.

We can all do more, and if we want to see change, we all *must* do more.

WHAT YOU'LL FIND INSIDE AND HOW TO GET THE MOST FROM IT

This book is shaped around my personal journey of the past four years; it's the story of what I've learned from that day in January 2018 that changed my life for ever.

Please be advised: Chapter 2 is a description of my experiences of the night Sam died. After reading this Introduction, and particularly the section on how necessary uncomfortable conversations are, I hope you understand why I have chosen to tell that story. I feel it is essential for us not to continue to skirt around the crux of these issues. What I describe actually happened to me and it is happening to other people right *now*. My hope is that reading about that night will help those who have gone through something similar, those who may suspect someone they know feels the same way Sam did, and those who want a better understanding of what it all means.

Within the chapters you'll find fact boxes and strategies to help you navigate certain situations and become better informed on everything from grief, guilt and shame to CPR and the fight-or-flight response. I know there is *loads* of information out there about mental health, but I want this to be more intimate than just googling some resources. Read along, learn from my mistakes, and we can have a laugh and a cry together – and feel all the better for it. This book has been written for you. That's how personal it is: you're not reading a fictional tale, you're reading my life, plain and simple, in black and white.

One of the most profound things I've been told is: 'We are human beings, not human doings.' Sometimes the best, most effective thing is to simply *be*, not do. So, I ask that you please take a step back every so often while reading this book, look away and just let it sink in. Let your thoughts go wherever they want to go. I promise, if you can nail doing that and get good at just being present, it's better than drugs!

And finally, I should point out that there's no happily ever after to this story. In parts it might feel exhausting or overwhelming. That's okay. Just notice how you feel and take a break if you need to. Having said that, there is hope here. Yes, the situation is shit and I'm not going to paint it otherwise – but there are so many people out there trying to make it better every single day. We ARE making progress – the fact this book has even been published is testament to that. Not so long ago, pitching a book on the reality of suicide and the UK's mental health crisis would have got you laughed out of the building.

So while this book doesn't have a happily ever after, hopefully by the end we'll be one step closer to it.

Please note, some people's personal details have been changed in order to protect their identity.

CHAPTER 1

A NORMAL FAMILY

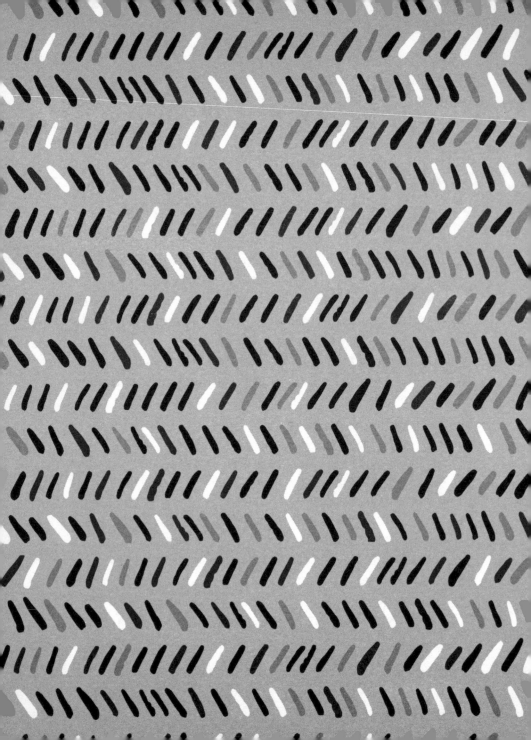

In proper Disney style, this story begins with a forest, a dog and a normal family. That warm fuzzy feeling you get at the start of fairy tales is exactly how I feel looking back on my childhood. But just because the story starts well, doesn't mean you're any less likely to meet a big bad wolf. That's why beginning here is so important.

I had a truly wonderful upbringing. My two brothers and I grew up with our mum, dad and collie-labrador, Tippy, in a small village in Kent called Frittenden. Kent is justifiably known as 'the Garden of England' with fields as far as the eye can see and acres of woodland to get lost in. It's also the birthplace of the sandwich, which is reason enough to rate the place.

We grew up in an old beautiful farmhouse smack-bang in the middle of nowhere, the sheep outnumbering people about ten to one. The house is quaint and lovely ... until spider season arrives. You'll look up and think, 'Why is that old oak beam moving?' And then, upon closer inspection, you realise that spiders are – and I use this word quite literally – *erupting* out of the woodwork. As someone who can't be in the same room as anything with more than four legs and two eyes, that's not ideal. But, house spiders aside, the house is great. It's like when you own an old car and everything that goes wrong isn't a problem but part of its character. For example, my bedroom window has never shut properly and we've always just accepted that as a fact. If it got fixed, the room wouldn't be the same.

The relative isolation of living somewhere like this means people grow very close to those around them, and that was definitely true of me and my brothers. We spent near enough all of our time together, either as friends or foes. I was two years older than Sam and four years older than Tom. As a baby, I was given all the love, uncontested, so you can bet I was pretty miffed when Sam came along and my parents' attention was suddenly shared. My mum tells me now that she used to put Sam down as a baby whenever I walked into the room to stop me from getting jealous. But, being the eldest – as I'm sure a few of you will relate to – does come with its perks. I got all the new clothes, which I then merrily passed on to my brothers full of holes, I got to try everything first, and I also got to sit in the front seat on school runs without ever having to call shotgun. To balance that out though, every accident or injury that befell any of us was automatically my fault, even if it was most definitely not my fault. For example, here's a story I'll never forget: for my tenth birthday, I had a go-karting party. All of my friends were coming over to the house before we left for the track, and while waiting for them to arrive, Sam, Tom and I decided to go on the trampoline in our garden. We bloody loved that thing! We'd bounce around, holding or throwing my mum's exercise ball at each other for added laughs.

And then Sam broke my ankle.

Yep, just as everyone was arriving for my party, Sam fell weirdly and landed on my ankle, and SNAP! I remember sitting in the corner of the kitchen as my friends turned up, my leg balanced on the table, an ice pack on my ankle. My dad being my dad picked me up saying, 'It's fine! You can walk on that!' Safe to say, I definitely couldn't. My mum and I ended up spending the next six hours in Maidstone Hospital A&E, while all of my friends went go-karting with my dad ... and Sam. Because, of course, he took my place. Cheeky fucker. We used to laugh about that a lot. And, of course, me being the eldest, we all agreed it was probably my fault anyway.

Another vivid memory I have of my childhood stars Tom. He had this weird thing when he was young where he would faint randomly – suddenly keel over like those goats in the viral YouTube videos that pass out when they're shocked. So, *obviously*, Sam and I used to surprise him ALL THE TIME, rolling around in hysterics when he hit the deck unconscious. Looking back on it, the fact he fainted like that was probably quite serious. I do remember that my mum certainly didn't find it funny. But hell, I won't lie to you – it was fucking funny to me and Sam. (Un)fortunately Tom grew out of whatever that was, eventually becoming less of a goat and more a fully functioning human; great for him, but a massive shame for me and Sam.

PLAYING PIRATES IN SCILLY

We used to go on family holidays to the Isles of Scilly, just off the coast of Cornwall, pretty much every year. Twenty-six miles off Land's End, they are an archipelago of islands that genuinely look like the tropical paradise islands you get on picture postcards: tranquil turquoise seas lapping against soft sandy beaches.

Bryher, one of the islands, is without doubt one of my favourite places on the planet. Tom, Sam and I would spend hours in the sea there – which, by the way, may *look* tropical but definitely doesn't *feel* tropical – dragging each other under the waves and screaming when the ice-cold water entered our wetsuits. We'd spend whole days on the beach, burying each other under the sand, then running off and leaving whoever was stuck there. We'd also hire a small boat from the local boatyard, and drive to different islands, anchor up and pretend we were pirates. (Yes, the type of pirates who'd bring their parents along and have picnics on the beach, but pirates nonetheless.)

Scilly was a place where we could be wild and feral and free.

As we grew up, we started working summer seasons on the islands. When I was 13, I started working for that same Bryher boatyard – Hut 62 as it's now known – spending as much time as possible stretching the concept of 'work' to breaking point by driving the boats across the mirror-flat turquoise sea in the sun. Of course, the boss would have something to say about that as there was plenty of other stuff to do – stuff that would leave you bruised and knackered – but I loved that just as much. Meanwhile, Sam worked for the island's hotel, brilliantly named after its location: Hell Bay Hotel. He also used to sell handmade model sailing boats that he'd crafted out of driftwood from a stall on the side of the road (well, less a 'road', more a dirt track for the four or five cars on the whole island). And he'd sell loads! People couldn't get enough of them. They weren't just taking pity on the kid – the models were actually good; he was an incredibly talented artist.

God, we really loved those times. Looking back now, I'm really grateful we got to share those trips.

TEENAGE KICKS

As teenagers, perhaps unsurprisingly, my relationship with my brothers changed. I'm sure everyone who's also grown up with siblings of a similar age will relate when I say: you know *exactly* how to get on each other's nerves. And there's no better way of doing that than deciding you want to learn to play the bloody trumpet, like Sam did. Is there anything worse than a kid learning to play the trumpet? Oh yes, a kid learning to play the drums. That'd be Tom. And then there was me, who, not to be outdone, decided to learn the saxophone. Can you even imagine what our house must have sounded like? How on earth my parents, or the sheep outside, coped is a mystery.

Credit where credit's due though: Sam did get better. (And, oh boy, were we all relieved when he did!) Truth was, he was just as talented at music as he was at art. I laugh at the memory of him honking through trumpet practice now, when in reality he picked it up very quickly. And then Sam moved on to the piano ... and, when he was about 13 years old, he started *composing his own music digitally*. He loved Hans Zimmer – the composer of some of the best-known Hollywood movie scores ever. For his GCSE music project he produced his own version of 'Time', that famous tune from the film *Inception*.

You know the one that goes: *dah duh duh duh daaah*. Hmm, okay, turns out it's difficult to describe on paper, but it's far harder to reproduce digitally, I'd imagine. How on earth do you even start to do that?!

I have to confess that I did use to make fun of his music taste: Classic FM was certainly not my vibe. But I can see why he liked it and appreciated it. It's funny because now I find myself listening to classical music a lot more. There's something really beautiful and serene about it. Plus, it makes me feel important and sophisticated having a cello concerto playing in the background over dinner. Fake it until you make it, right?

As well as crafting models and making music, Sam could paint. Some of the landscapes he painted were really quite remarkable. A mix of both abstract and realism. There wouldn't necessarily be anything obvious like a tree or a house; more a suggestion of form. In fact, right now as I'm writing this, I'm looking at one of his paintings hanging on the wall: it shows the silhouette of a hill drowning in a burning red sunset. It's simultaneously bleak and simple, while exploding in colour and detail. I really don't think his paintings would look out of place in a gallery. Not only that, but I think they would be some of the best stuff in that gallery.

I didn't share Sam's gift for the arts – that gene blew straight past me. I was okay at music, if by okay you mean making a noise and being able to vaguely hold a rhythm. But my painting skills were – and still are – atrocious. So, while Sam was out there creating spot-on homages of famous artists' work, I was having to start again because I'd coloured over the lines. I also just didn't have the patience for it. I get bored far too easily. I won't say no to watching an episode of *The Joy of Painting with Bob Ross* though. (I'll level with you, I wasn't expecting Bob Ross to make a cameo in my book, but hey, welcome to the story, Bob.) So, while Sam was working to become either the next Bob Ross (there he is again, sorry) or Hans Zimmer, I was spending my time outside in and among the trees. Actually often *up* the trees. My hobby was running about in nature, totally carefree. It probably sounds a bit odd, but looking back I can't think of much else I did. Maybe it's time I had a conversation with my mum and dad about the possibility that I was adopted from the rainforest and had my tail removed.

This disparity in pastimes definitely contributed to Sam and I drifting apart, and I noticed it. My making fun of his interests probably didn't help. And no, I'm not proud of that. If you find something interesting or fun, if you enjoy it, then that's your right and no one should have any say over it. No one should judge you. But we do judge, right? I guess I might have been a bit jealous that he had hobbies he was not only really good at, but also really passionate about.

All of this made the times when we did get on even better though. And some of the best times we ever had were during Christmas when we'd join forces to terrorise my grandmother (my dad's mum), Yvett, from whom Sam definitely inherited his artistic talent. Yvett is flipping hilarious, full of such great stories, and we'd always look forward to seeing her – and to winding her up. Sam, Tom and I made it our goal to give her the most outrageous Christmas gifts just to see her reaction:

classics included a unicorn onesie and a dot-to-dot book of naked male strippers, some with whips and others … Well, let's just say, they were 'enjoying themselves'.

The absolute highlight though, which had us laughing for years, was the year we got her (fake) tickets to do a skydive with a friend. She was 80 years old. You should have seen the look on her face! Priceless. Best of all though, she didn't want to seem ungrateful so she accepted the tickets with a big smile and a lot of thanks. A couple of hours later, my mum (who was in on the joke) pulled me aside and said, 'Grandma's just told me that she's really worried she doesn't think she'd be able to do a skydive because of her knees.' Absolutely golden. Of course, my grandma being my grandma, when she did eventually find out it was a joke, decided to pay the laughs forward and convinced her friends it was real and asked them to come with her. She was in stitches telling us that. So yes, I can attest that Christmas is definitely all about the 'gift of giving' – the gift of giving my grandma terrible presents and getting a lot of laughs in return.

And that's what Sam and I *did* have in common: we loved a good laugh. Whether it was a prank, a joke or some general silliness, Sam was not only very funny, he also had an infectious chuckle. Sometimes, when you worked out why he was laughing, even if the joke made you cringe and was seriously close to crossing a line, the fact *he* found it so funny would make you crack up nevertheless.

That's what I noticed most significantly when he started to get older – the laughing stopped. From the age of 15, he started becoming much quieter, especially over dinner. Whereas previously he'd always been loud and fun around the table, telling stories about his day and his friends, it was like he'd suddenly run out of things to say. He also stopped asking questions. And yeah, we've all been there – tired after a long day and not in the mood to talk or have a joke. Yet this wasn't a one-off, it was every day. He'd be there, in the room, but also not there at all.

At the time, this really annoyed me. Partly, I think, because for so long I'd really enjoyed his personality and was therefore really sad that it had changed. But also because I found his new attitude irritating. He would constantly sigh, only respond to questions with one-word answers, not make eye contact or even look up from his plate. The longer this went on, the more I started to lose patience with him. His mood affected the whole family. It's hard for anyone else to have a chat or a laugh when there's someone at the table who clearly doesn't want to be there.

Looking back now, it's obvious that something was going on. It's brazenly evident that he wasn't okay. But hindsight's 20/20, isn't it? Because at the time, I just thought he was being moody. What 15-year-old wants to play happy families every night at dinner? I know I sure didn't when I was 15. But then again – I did sometimes. I really used to enjoy our evenings together. Sure, I would have off-days, but I'd also have on-days. Days when I would want to engage and muck about and get involved. Sam never did – and yet, he seemed okay at school. I'd see him seemingly having a good time with his mates, so it was just at home that he clammed up. And that made me mad because it became about *us*, his family. It seemed as though he didn't like *us*. And after a while, that does get to you – the thought that this might be about you. You get defensive. We weren't so bad! It wasn't fair that his friends always got 'fun' Sam and we always got 'grumpy' Sam.

I genuinely didn't think anything was actually *wrong*; I just thought he was in a permanent teenage strop with us and that he needed to snap out of it. It didn't cross my mind that he might be putting on a mask with his friends and that he actually felt safe and comfortable enough at home to show his true feelings around us.

A DIAGNOSIS AND A MISUNDERSTANDING

One night after dinner in September 2017, when Sam had been acting the way described above for a fair few months, I was sitting on the AGA in the kitchen chatting to my mum. (I always used to sit on the AGA in winter. I'd put a towel over the top of it and then sit half on, half off, so one side of me would be really warm.) So, I was sitting there, happily getting an AGA tan, when my mum turned around and suddenly said, 'Sam has been diagnosed with clinical depression.' My face went blank. That meant nothing to me. I remember thinking, 'What on earth is depression? How can you be diagnosed with "being sad"? Also, why is Mum telling me this like it's some sort of a big deal? Just go out, see your friends and be happy? Right?'

If she'd said cancer I would have certainly reacted differently. I would have understood the seriousness of it. I would have known that meant that Sam was ill and would need treatment. That this would affect his life and our lives and that it should be taken seriously.

But she didn't. She said depression.

DEPRESSION: THE LOW-DOWN

Experiencing sadness for a bit is totally normal. The feeling will pass and you'll feel other emotions again – including happiness and joy. But what if those feelings don't pass? When you're depressed you experience persistent low mood and sadness and/or a marked loss of interest or pleasure. Depression can be categorised into varying levels: mild, moderate and severe.

Symptoms of depression include:

* feelings of worthlessness or excessive or inappropriate guilt;
* disturbed sleep (decreased or increased compared to usual);
* decreased or increased appetite and/or weight;
* fatigue or loss of energy;
* agitation or slowing of movements;

»

* poor concentration or indecisiveness;
* suicidal thoughts or acts.

If you have five of the above symptoms you may be suffering with mild depression, more than five can indicate moderate depression, while experiencing *all* of the symptoms – to the point where they affect your ability to function within your normal life – suggests you might be suffering from severe, or clinical, depression.[1]
Depression is one of the most common forms of mental illness, with more than 264 million people suffering from it around the world.[2] Nearly 20 per cent of people in the UK aged 16 and over show symptoms of anxiety or depression.[3]

If you think you, or someone you know, might have depression, you should contact a GP as they'll be able to assess the symptoms and discuss options going forward. Seeking help is really important because the right support, especially early on, increases the chances of recovery.

WHY DO PEOPLE GET DEPRESSION?

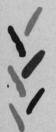

Lots of factors can affect the likelihood of someone suffering from depression, including brain chemistry, genetic predisposition, social and environmental factors, life changes, stressors, and individual personality traits (i.e. your belief in your ability to cope). Sometimes depression can be triggered by a life event, but generally it's caused by a combination of things. Here I'd like to explain a little about the role that your brain chemistry plays, which means we need to talk about neurotransmitters, neurons and hormones. If you aren't a fan of long words and biology, please bear with me; I'll try my best to make this interesting.

You're no doubt familiar with the term 'brain cells' – the cells that give the brain the ability to do its job. They're also known as neurons or nerve cells. These cells communicate with each other via signals that can send nerve impulses throughout your body. Signals can be sent to muscles to create movement or to glands to release hormones, and loads of other fancy things. Also, within your brain and around all the cells are chemicals called neurotransmitters. Their job is to help carry, boost and balance the nerve signals travelling through the network of cells. They are REALLY important. Billions of neurotransmitter molecules are in your brain right now enabling it to function. You know how you just took a breath? That's down to cells, signals and neurotransmitters.

The key thing with neurotransmitters, though, is that they can affect your emotions. Ever done something that's made you feel really good? (I know what you're thinking – behave.) That's because more of the neurotransmitter dopamine has been released. Ever done something that's really stressed you out? (Watched Spurs lose in the eighty-seventh minute, am I right?!) That'll be the chemical cortisol being released. Ever felt all warm and buzzy, like you're in love? That'll be the oxytocin.

Research has found that the science of feelings – what triggers your emotional responses – is, to a certain extent, controlled by the concentration of neurotransmitters in your brain. Mental illnesses

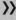

(as well as some physical conditions) can therefore also be, to a similar extent, affected or caused by imbalances of neuro-transmitters. A few things that might cause these imbalances are:

- Neurons not manufacturing enough of a particular neurotransmitter.
- Neurotransmitters being reabsorbed back into the neuron too quickly.
- Too many neurotransmitters being deactivated by enzymes.
- Too much of a particular neurotransmitter being released.

Lots of different things might trigger these problems. For example, it might be a hormonal issue, as hormones directly affect neurotransmitters – particularly serotonin, dopamine and norepinephrine – which is why you see an increase in mood fluctuations during times when your hormones are changing, i.e. during periods, pregnancy or puberty. It can even be from brain trauma, the result of an illness or an accident.

People can find mental illness difficult to understand or picture, which is why understanding the role brain chemistry might play can really help. If your neurotransmitters aren't functioning at the optimum levels, you'll likely feel changes in mood. Sure, this is a highly simplified explanation (I could get *deep* into chat about 'axon terminals' and 'gamma-aminobutyric acid', but, to be honest, I'd rather sing you a song while dressed as Robin Hood (see page 47), so please trust me when I say that this is the crux of it).

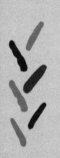

Please note though: brain science is endlessly debated as it's so complex (I always think brain research is weird because essentially it's brains learning about themselves), so there will always be new research, as well as newly developed and disputed theories. However, I believe acknowledging that hormones play a massive part in emotions is a really important part of the mental health conversation because it makes mental illnesses more understandable to many and so less stigmatised.

I definitely knew about the phrase 'mental health'. We'd been told about it at school, for sure. I think we'd even had a couple of outside speakers do an assembly or two on the subject. But I'd always clocked out because: emotions? Gross. Super-awkward to talk about. Especially as a boy – being emotional, affectionate or vulnerable was something I didn't see as okay. This belief went so deep that I never even hugged my friends, and my friendship group was very huggy. I'd just get a hug and not reciprocate, standing there awkwardly with my hands by my sides. It didn't feel like a manly thing to do. There, I said it: 'manly'. Urg. But where the hell had that come from? How had that belief infiltrated my mindset? Was it from films, books, TV, society, culture, history, music? All of the above? I don't know, but it certainly impacted on me. I remember so clearly wanting to put up this front, to act like I didn't care, like I was a tough guy. Who was I kidding?!

Believing that contributed to the way I shrugged off Sam's diagnosis – on top of the fact that I genuinely did think depression was a minor thing. Me, being the default-positive, always-look-on-the-bright-side, glass-half-full, playing-the-glad-game kinda guy I am, thought that my mum had essentially just revealed that Sam was 'a bit down'. And we all feel like that sometimes, don't we, so how bad could it be?

One thing that did stick with me though, was when my mum then told me that Sam didn't want me to know. She said she was telling me because she thought I should be aware of what was going on, but that he had told her not to tell me. I remember that stung a bit, but again, I didn't think too much about it. At the end of the day, that was fair enough, I reasoned. His life, his business. Who was I to know everything about it? No one, that's who.

Sam did find out that my mum had told me though and he didn't like it *at all*. From my perspective, looking back, I now think that he was ashamed of his diagnosis and embarrassed about people knowing. So he was dealing now not only with depression and anxiety, but also with shame and probably guilt – two of the worst emotions in the world (more on them on page 97).

Every so often my mum gave me updates. But, to be honest, my memory is a little hazy about these because they seemed really insignificant to me at the time. And that's the truth. I thought Sam was sad, that's it. And so when my mum said, 'He's getting help', I was like, 'Great. Brill. Top-drawer' and went on my way – because what else was I supposed to think or do? Again, I didn't know what 'getting help' meant, so I left everyone else to it. I remember at one point she told me that Sam 'didn't like CBT [Cognitive Behavioural Therapy] and didn't think it was working', but – and you'll have started noticing a pattern here – I didn't understand it, so I didn't take much notice.

As much as these mini-updates were about Sam, a part of me can't help but wonder now if they were also a chance for my mum to get things off her chest. While she obviously spoke to my dad about it, Sam didn't. Sam didn't talk to anyone about any of it except Mum and a couple of his close friends. So she took it all on. She took him to counselling, she investigated help, she worried about his schoolwork, his friends and his health. She was his sounding board and Sam had been adamant that no one else was to know. She must have felt very alone in it. And the rest of the family didn't know what to do. We thought we were doing the right thing by abiding by his wishes. I can't imagine how stressful that time was for Mum. I don't know why I didn't see it at the time. Why didn't I realise what was going on? If only I'd have taken more notice. But then again, sometimes we turn a blind eye to things *not* because we don't understand or don't recognise that they're bad, but because we don't want to concede that something is wrong. We don't *want* something to be wrong. Maybe my not taking it seriously was as much about not *wanting* to understand as it was about not actually understanding. It was safer not knowing. The Sam that I grew up with, the Sam that was brilliant to be around, wasn't there any more. Perhaps I didn't want to accept that, so instead I just became annoyed about it.

I wonder.

I never spoke to him about it. Not once, ever. We never even acknowledged it. Siblings hate each other one minute and love each other the next, but no matter what, you're there for them if they need help. If Sam or Tom were getting bullied, or if someone was giving them shit, I'd like to think I'd have stood up for them. I actually never had to – so that's a good thing, I think? That protectiveness is instinct though; you can't remove it. And it's probably even stronger when you're the eldest. When I argued with Sam and Tom, I felt awful about upsetting them. My words and actions always made me feel worse than they ever did them. I've always been like that: an emotional sponge. I'll absorb other people's emotions and if they hurt, I

SOMETIMES WE TURN A BLIND EYE TO THINGS NOT BECAUSE WE DON'T UNDERSTAND OR DON'T RECOGNISE THAT THEY'RE BAD, BUT BECAUSE WE DON'T WANT TO CONCEDE THAT SOMETHING IS WRONG.

hurt. Empathy's a big thing with me. I've always had a sense of when things were becoming uncomfortable for someone and mirrored their discomfort internally.

That's why, looking back, it's incredibly confusing and hard to acknowledge how casual I was about Sam's situation. Did I not understand or did I not want to understand? I don't know.

TIPS FOR HELPING SOMEONE WHO'S STRUGGLING

LEARN TO LISTEN

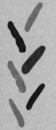

People won't talk if there's no one willing to hear them. And, while everyone acknowledges how important it is to open up, far fewer people understand the power of giving their time to simply listen.

If you suspect someone is struggling then assume that you're the only one who does. Reach out, send a text, call them, invite them for coffee, ask them how they are, give them the space to talk. I know in practice it's so much easier said than done. Fuck – look at my story. I knew Sam was struggling and never asked him about it. Why? There are loads of reasons:

* It's natural to assume that things are actually 'not that bad'.
* No one wants to focus on the worst-case scenario so will default to the best case.
* We all have our own shit to deal with.
* We're scared of things we don't understand.
* It's easier to think someone else will handle it – and they'll handle it better than we will.
* It strikes a painful chord within our own lives that we don't want to acknowledge.
* The conversation is daunting as hell. I mean, it's not going to be a laugh-riot, is it?

My advice? Act now and think later. Sending a text can be a great way of starting that conversation. Here are some example messages to send to someone you're worried about:

* 'Hey mate, have noticed you don't seem yourself at the moment. Do you want to talk about anything?'
* 'Roses are red, feeling sad sucks, just want you to know, that I give a fuck. Lol that sounded better in my head, but seriously, I'm here if you need to chat.'
* 'Just wanted to say, I have *[whatever they're going through]* and so I know how tough it is. Hope you're doing okay.'
* 'Totally okay if you don't want to respond, I won't take it personally, but I'm here if you ever want to process some stuff.'
* 'Just wanted to let you know I'm thinking of you. If you ever need someone to swing by, I'd love to.'

»

SELF-CARE STRATEGIES FOR DEPRESSION

As much as it's important to check in with others, it's arguably even more so to look after yourself. Here are some starter strategies to try yourself.

TALKING

If you have depression or are struggling with your emotions, there are lots of things you can do to try to feel better. The first thing, though, should absolutely be: talk about it. Even if you don't think it's anything serious, if you find your mood is affecting your day-to-day life, speaking to someone about it is really important. Chat to a family member, a friend, your GP or an anonymous helpline (please see page 281).

Please know that there is treatment available that can help to make you feel better.

Beyond talking, there are also a whole host of good practices that can help you to feel better and protect you from feeling worse. Some of the suggestions here may sound inconsequential – you may even think that bringing them up is trivialising what you're going through – but small actions really can make a big impact.

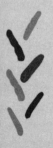

MINDFULNESS

Mindfulness is a word that's bounced around a lot – and that's because it's a powerful tool if used properly. In essence, mindfulness is bringing your attention completely to the present moment. Learning how to tune into your body and your thoughts so you can interrupt negative patterns. It's about engaging your senses and snapping out of autopilot: what can you hear, see, smell, touch and taste? What are your thoughts doing right now? It's about being non-judgemental and compassionate to yourself: not berating yourself for how you're thinking, but just *noticing* it. Then you're giving yourself a choice if you want to continue down those paths.

Mindfulness also helps you to get a better sense of how your body influences your mind and vice versa. If your shoulders are hunched and your fists clenched, how does that make you feel emotionally? And does dropping your shoulders, unclenching your fists and putting your chin up make you feel calmer?

There are lots of books and resources available online that'll teach you about mindfulness if you want to learn more. There are also people who can teach you how to do this either as part of a group or one-on-one. I recommend researching the most popular apps to start with. Headspace and Calm are good for a bit of zen.

PHYSICAL HEALTH

Don't underestimate the importance of physical health on your mental health. I always find it strange how we separate the two

››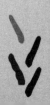

when they're one and the same. Fitness and nutrition play major roles in helping to prevent mental illness as well as aiding recovery. We've discussed how mental illness is related to neurotransmitters and hormones, in particular identifying dopamine, norepinephrine and serotonin, as crucial to mood – well, guess which hormones are released during exercise? Yep. Regular exercise has even been shown to have the opposite effect on the brain as depression.[4, 5]

Although self-care is not the magic solution to mental illness, it can help. Once again though, I'll reiterate, if your mood is affecting you day-to-day and you have symptoms of mental illness, getting advice from a professional is really important.

■

GREEN BANANAS

When I was super-young, I was also super-sensitive. One day, when I was about eight years old, the teacher blew the whistle to signal the end of break and I cried because it was too loud. But, as I got older, I started to feel safer and became more outgoing and more confident. More myself. When I was 10, I ran for Head of House and won by a landslide because Sam got his whole year to vote for me! Thanks Sam, appreciate that one. Get me: Head of Leeds House at Sutton Valence Prep (big up). Hardly seems like much looking back on it, but at the time I felt great. I really loved primary school. To be honest, I probably didn't learn much, but I had a laugh and it was genuinely just a great place to be. Hell, I was even Robin Hood in our Year 6 play and had to sing a song[6]. Hang on, here goes:

> *Forever friends we will be*
> *Like a pair of forest trees*
> *Side by side 'till the end*
> *We will be forever friends.*

Ha! I still remember it! There's actually a video somewhere of me singing that song and I'm going to try my absolute hardest to ensure it never resurfaces. That performance epitomises that period of my life though – I didn't care what anyone thought, and I excelled in myself and as myself.

The academic side was, um, not so good ... but who cared?! I mean, apart from my parents and all the teachers. In hindsight, yes, maybe I could have done with a little more direction. I do have a vivid memory of getting detention for eating a glue 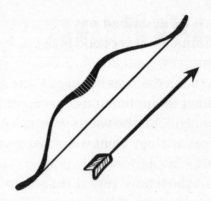 stick. (I'm pretty sure I was fed at home, so I have no idea where that urge came from.) And yes, okay, as I've already mentioned, my English skills weren't the best. I was told I had to skip French classes so I could attend extra English lessons one-on-one with a nice teacher called Mrs Faulkner. Ah, bless Mrs Faulkner and her unlimited patience. My spelling and grammar was so atrocious that it was lucky my name was as simple as Ben, otherwise my work would have been anonymous. As mentioned in the Introduction, at the end of my time at primary school my parents were told that it would be best if I didn't sit the 11-plus exams as 'it will be demoralising for him'. Imagine that! The school was so convinced that I'd fail, they told me not to even bother turning up. I did feel pretty deflated watching everyone go off, nervously clutching their pencils and chewed biros, while I was left in a room with a handful of people who couldn't use commas correctly. (I'm still not very, good, at punctuation, though, I, can't; lie.) The school described me as 'a green banana' in my final report. Hmm. It's never good being likened to an unripe piece of fruit. But, yes, I might have been a green banana, albeit a green banana that was having the time of its life as part of a bunch of other green bananas – some of whom I'm still in touch with today. And who wants to be ripe at 11 years old anyway? (Okay, that analogy went weird really quickly. Apologies. Blame my old school.)

School was very different for Sam, even though he had a lovely group of friends. I think he found it difficult to fit in and questioned what exactly his place or 'role' was. Many people can probably relate to how having a herd, a group to call your own, as well as a certainty and confidence in your place within that herd, is really powerful. If you don't have it, you can feel cut adrift. I've always found it fairly easy to fit in anywhere, and when you do, you don't realise how hard it can be for other people. One of the most devastating things I have learned through my campaigning is just how many people feel lonely, especially young people. I was involved in a study by Accenture during the pandemic which suggested that 55 per cent[7] of university students felt lonely either every day or every week. Loneliness is a dark place and can be incredibly damaging. I wouldn't cope very well with feeling lonely. Not to have companionship or support – or to think that you don't (or can't) have it – is awful.

When Sam was diagnosed he really wanted people to understand mental health. Of the two of us, he was the first to start campaigning. He actually made anonymous posters that he put up around the school about the subject. I remember seeing them everywhere, but had no idea he'd made them, until I found one in his bag at home. It read – and I remember this clear as day – 'Depression is feeling alone but not wanting anyone to be around.' That hit me hard. It still does. It was such an insight into his mindset at the time and strikes right at the heart of what I think are some of the most important things we have in life: companionship, a sense of belonging, and a sense of self-worth. Sam wanted people to understand and wanted things to change so he didn't have to feel so ashamed and suppressed. Like I said though, he did have friends and they were incredible, but his illness took away the joy in that.

Depression is so complicated. There's no one-size-fits-all. There's no rulebook – for either those suffering or those who love them. I wish there had been, because maybe what happened next, wouldn't have. But who knows? I can only hope that if, having read this far, any of this strikes a chord, you'll read on, because it may help. You may recognise what Sam went through or what I went through. Before that though, please do have a cup of tea, go for a walk, and get ready, because Chapter 2's a big one.

DEPRESSION IS FEELING ALONE BUT NOT WANTING ANYONE TO BE AROUND.

TAKEAWAYS

- Depression is an illness, not a weakness, and not the result of anything anyone has done 'wrong'. Recognising this is immensely important as a step towards greater understanding and compassion.

- Remember: we all wear masks and neither suffering with depression nor loving someone who does is easy – but pretending that nothing is happening will make things harder. Learning, talking and listening are good first steps.

- If you're feeling down and it's starting to affect your day-to-day life then talking to someone is really important. Please reach out to a friend, family member, GP or helpline.

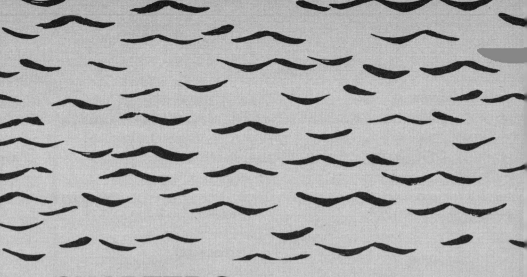

CHAPTER 2
21/01/2018

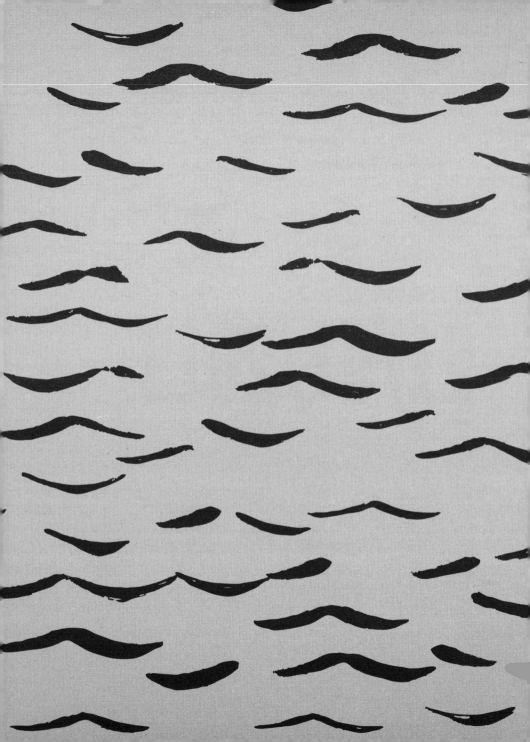

Perhaps unsurprisingly, when you're writing a book, you start to think about life in terms of chapters. Different periods of time or certain events that shape your story. Perhaps more unusual though, is when you realise that one of those chapters will need to come with a warning. This is such a chapter and here's the warning: what follows is a description of suicide that may be upsetting or triggering for some readers.

The truth is that none of what is described here was expected or predicted by anyone involved. The harrowing nature of mental illness is that, when it wins, it's sudden, unexpected and unbearable.

When I was young I'd sometimes think about what a future book of my life might include: where I'd go, who I'd meet and what I'd do. It excited me. All the possibilities, all the stories! I didn't ever imagine I'd actually get to write one, let alone while I was still so young – and I certainly didn't imagine that it would be inspired by the following pages.

My brother, Sam, loved life. He *loved* it. Life filled his art, his camera lens and his dreams. He always said he wanted to go to Canada one day to experience the epic scenery and 'be among the vastness of life'. I find myself thinking about him whenever I watch the sunrise or hear the birds singing in the morning. I think about him when I see a fox run into the hedgerows. I think about him when I hear the roar of water-falls and rivers. I think about him when I watch the sky catch on fire at sunset. I think about him as the stars and moon fill every inch of the night sky. I think about him in every frame of beauty this planet has to offer.

But while Sam loved *life* – he didn't like his.

Just before writing this, I flicked through Sam's art book. It's stunning; he was so talented. But by far the most striking part for me is not the quality of his work, but the fact that it just stops midway through. There's a positive note from his teacher on a drawing . . . and then just a whole bunch of empty pages. I can't help but wonder what might have filled those pages, how he might have illustrated the chapters of his own life in that book. I wonder where he'd go, who he'd meet and what he'd do. I can't help but wonder what he could have become.

Inevitably this chapter is extremely distressing, and, if you think you'll find it triggering, I would encourage you to skip ahead to Chapter 3.

All too often we talk about suicide as an abstract thing – something that happens to other people or is reeled out as a sad statistic. Suicide has become accepted as just another tragic inevitability of life. But what happened to Sam and what happened to my family *is* something that needs to be told. We can't brush over the reality of what it means to experience suicide if we want to find ways to try to prevent it, as well as to help those who go through what my family did. It ties back into what I said in the Introduction: we *must* be willing to have both the pretty and the ugly conversations.

This will likely be a tough read – it's uncomfortable, raw and emotional. But, I didn't read this in a book, I lived it. In fact, I still live it every single day. Suicide is not something we should ever just accept; it is an event in which one person loses their life and hundreds of other people's lives shatter to pieces. We

I WONDER WHERE HE'D GO, WHO HE'D MEET AND WHAT HE'D DO. I CAN'T HELP BUT WONDER WHAT HE COULD HAVE BECOME.

must do absolutely everything we can to try to prevent it if possible, and acknowledging the actuality of the experience is a necessary part of that process.

So yes, this chapter will be hard to read, but that's why it's so important it exists.

A BROKEN RIB AND THE WINTER BLUES

The year 2018 introduced itself to me in a way that pretty much summed up what it would bring: it started with me falling on some ice and breaking a rib in my back. (Yes, this is the second time that I've started a story with me breaking a bone and we're only on Chapter 2. And guess what? It won't be the last . . .)

Our family had been skiing and snowboarding over the New Year. Us three boys were at about the same skill level, so we'd often go off together. Tom and I were snowboarders while Sam would 'stick to skis, thank you very much'. So Tom and I would be tearing up powder and jumping over crests while Sam clinically and efficiently made his way down the slopes.

One morning, we were going down a black run that was very steep and icy. I won't try and big myself up here: the truth is that I just ran out of talent, slipping and falling backwards onto the ice. I knocked my head and winded myself, but that's standard when snowboarding, so I didn't think much of it as I wasn't in much pain – my pride was hurt more than anything else. I got up, shook myself off and boarded back down the piste. It was only at the bottom that I noticed the dull ache in my back; it felt like a trapped nerve. I asked my dad if he could try to release it so I stood in the middle of a crowd, throwing shapes, while he twisted and massaged my shoulder. It was uncomfortable, but not painful, so I carried on snowboarding for the rest of the week.

The moment we returned home though, it all went wrong. As I took my shirt off to get into the shower, CRACK! My rib split in two. I'd actually fractured it during the fall and taking my shirt off had pulled it apart. Ouch. Not fancying another trip to A&E, I put a towel between my teeth to muffle my groans and got into the shower. I was soon busted though when Tom, hearing the squawking noises coming from my room as I tried to get into bed, told my mum he thought something must be wrong. Off to A&E we went. This injury particularly sucked because anyone who knows me knows how impossible I find it to go any length of time without having a laugh – and laughing with broken ribs is not the dream. Every breath was excruciating and each giggle would turn into a mixture of laugh-crying, me pleading with people to please stop being funny.

So 2018 was already pretty shit what with laughter physically hurting, A-Levels looming and having to write a bullshit personal statement about how I'd dreamed my whole life of attending university to study some course I had zero interest in. On top of that, I'm not a fan of British winters in general as they're dark, cold and miserable. In fact, I hate them so much, I often joke that I'll move somewhere hot, like California or Australia, given the opportunity. And I might really do that one day, for a winter or two (I'd just need to seriously assess the Australia spider situation). However, things perked up on 20 January when I got to go to Silverstone, driving high-performance Renaults with my dad. I loved that. My ribs didn't love it, but sod 'em – it was worth it, even if I did end up back in bed that night biting my towel.

Then Sunday 21 January arrived in classic British winter fashion: drizzly, cold and grey. Not cold enough to snow or warm enough to be interesting, just a nothing day. I did some school work in the afternoon and then, in the evening, after my dad had left to catch a train to London for work, my mum, Tom, Sam and I sat down for a meal.

21 JANUARY

At this point, I had become so used to Sam not engaging at dinner that I didn't think much of his silence. Yet, for some reason, that night felt different. The atmosphere was charged. It's impossible to explain, but it's like we all knew there was something clearly wrong. I remember Mum had made kebabs and they were delicious ... Yet Sam was entirely absent. He was there, but not, if that makes sense. And I found his attitude frustrating. So frustrating that I let him know about it. We had an argument and he stormed off.

I followed him upstairs shortly after he left the kitchen. I jumped in the shower, packed my bag for school the next day and then lay on my bed with my headphones on listening to some music. It was about 9.20 p.m. and Rudimental's *Not Giving In* was playing. During trauma there are some memories that remain sharp and fully focused, and the exact time and song I was listening to are ingrained in my mind. I heard my mum come upstairs to the first floor (the floor my room was on), and then head up one more flight to Sam's room in the attic. There was a short pause ... and then a scream shattered the quiet.

That sound echoes around my head even now as I sit here writing this. If you've never heard a scream of pure shock and horror before, you can't imagine it. It was a shriek that tore through my body and ignited every muscle. I ripped the headphones off and ran out of my room. I thought maybe she'd fallen over and cut herself on something. The run from my room to Sam's must be less than five seconds, but it felt like minutes. Like I was running in slow motion. The raw panic that had been bubbling up within me exploded as Mum started shouting my name. When I opened the door to Sam's room, I was faced with one of the most horrific things anyone could see: Sam had taken his own life.

I stood there for a few seconds, waiting for my brain to catch up to my eyes. Waiting for it to process what it was seeing. When something is so out of context, so shocking, it can seem as though you're watching a film. But that really did only last a second or two, because then it was like my body went into primitive survival mode. Autopilot switched on and started controlling what I did. It was entirely instinctual. I picked Sam up – even though he was a pretty big guy, it was as if he weighed nothing – and carried him over to an area of floor with more room and started CPR, which I'd learned at school in first aid courses.

Mum had run downstairs to grab her phone so she could call an ambulance. You may remember me describing how we lived in the middle of nowhere. Well, I think I speak for everyone that has ever needed an ambulance when I say you could live in the middle of central London and still feel like you're a million miles away from anyone and everything when you're on your knees waiting for help to arrive. When you're desperate for someone who knows what they're doing to take over.

My mum quickly came back with a 999 call handler on loudspeaker. To this day, the memory of hearing a tinny voice say, 'Listen to me very carefully; I'm going to talk you through resuscitation', sends shivers down my spine.

I'd always had an interest in becoming a paramedic one day, so had read a lot about pre-hospital care. What that meant was that I knew the chances of Sam surviving were very small. I knew that every pump I made that didn't cause him to breathe again was just further confirming that he was gone, and when his lips started turning blue I knew he wasn't coming back. Regardless though, I kept on. I kept being positive. I kept telling my mum that it would all be okay, that the ambulance would be here soon. Was I trying to reassure her or was I trying to reassure myself? I'm still not entirely sure.

'How long are you going to be? How long now? Are you nearly here?' I must have asked the call handler versions of that question a hundred times. And each time she responded, patiently and calmly, with, 'They're on their way. They're coming as quickly as they can.' And she was right. About fifteen minutes after I'd first opened Sam's door, we heard the faint sounds of sirens in the distance and I felt genuine bone-deep relief. So much so, that I actually laughed down the phone when I heard them. Can you believe it? The relief made me almost delirious. And then my mum started hyperventilating and I had to try to calm her down as well as continuing CPR. I thought she might be about to go into shock. The surrealness of the scene was too much and I remember saying to the woman on the phone, 'Now I have two patients', and laughing at the madness of it all. My mind had completely separated itself from reality. It was trying to make sense of a completely nonsensical situation; trying to find normalcy to ground me. My mum rushed downstairs to open the front door to flag down the ambulance and, about 20 minutes after I first started CPR, a man raced into the room wearing an official-looking green uniform. A paramedic was here! Thank God. 'Don't stop, keep going for me,' he said. 'I'm going to set up my kit and then take over, but keep going for now.'

To convey in any meaningful way the distress of trying to perform CPR on someone – on anyone, let alone someone you love – is incredibly difficult. I would not wish that situation on anybody. CPR is incredibly physically demanding. The force that you exert on the other person and therefore put your own body through is immense. That, on top of the emotional pressure of trying to process (or not process) what you're doing and why, makes the entire thing acutely physically and emotionally stressful. The only way I can even attempt to get across the trauma, is to remind you that I had a broken rib at the time. Anyone who has ever broken a bone knows how painful even the slightest movement can be. I did CPR for 20 minutes, with all the energy and strain focused on my back, lungs and arms, and I didn't notice a broken rib.

THIS ISN'T REAL; IT'S JUST THE WORST DREAM EVER

Leaving my mum and the paramedic with Sam, I went downstairs to check on Tom, knocking on his bedroom door and gently opening it. He was right behind the door as if he was expecting me. He looked shocked and confused and asked what was happening. I didn't know what to tell him, so I just said that there had been an accident. We went downstairs together and I sat him on the sofa in the living room and turned the TV on. I think *SpongeBob SquarePants* was showing. I closed the door, wanting to protect him as much as I could from seeing or knowing too much. He was only 13 years old.

After I'd made sure he was okay, I ran outside the house, onto the road, and started shouting at and waving down the emergency vehicles – of which there were at least six. A couple of ambulances, police cars, and even a fire engine. (A weird thing I recall – as I got to the road, an ambulance sped past the house and I tried to shout at it, but nothing came out. I couldn't make a sound. So, instead, I started clapping as loudly as I could to get the driver's attention.)

One thing I've always admired about paramedics is how they never look panicked, always projecting a cool, calm and collected vibe, even when with critical patients. Yet that night everything seemed speeded up. The Air Ambulance fast-response car shot past the house, before reversing and skidding right across our lawn, and the medical team leapt out in their orange flight suits almost before the car had come to a halt. They ran past me calling, 'Where do we go?' and I had to shout directions to their backs. That scene, more than any other, summed up how desperate and urgent this was. And then I was left watching the police, fire service personnel and paramedics swarming over the house, and I could see on their faces that they knew what was happening upstairs, that they'd been told, and that they were upset.

It wasn't just what I saw, it was also what I heard – a mix of voices, some shouting, some calm, all firm, the radios, alarms, doors slamming, weird bangs. It all became too much; I started shaking and my vision went blurry, my chest feeling tight. I felt faint and suddenly dropped to my knees and was violently sick in the nearby flower-bed. When I was able to get up, a paramedic rushed straight past me, not even checking to see if I was okay. That was another surreal moment in a list of many: it wouldn't actually be unusual to call an ambulance for someone who nearly passes out as they're being violently sick, yet here everyone rushed past me with bags of equipment, like I wasn't even there. That was very frightening – another punch-to-the-gut confirmation that what was happening to Sam was true. It was real. And it was really fucking serious. I wished they had stopped for me. I wished my situation had warranted concern because it would have meant that upstairs things weren't as bad as I'd seen.

So I stood there, looking at my driveway filled with all these strange and intimidating vehicles – vehicles that are never around for a good reason, that always herald bad news – with their harsh throbbing blue strobes, and I had a very strange moment.

None of this is real, I thought. *This is a bad dream.*

I genuinely believed that I was dreaming. One of those super-vivid nightmares that feel so real that Dream You can control what's happening. That was the only valid explanation my brain could come up with to process the trauma of what was happening. I was so convinced that it was a dream that I took out my phone and snapped a photo of all the chaos outside, totally sure that the photo would not be on my phone when I woke up. Taking that photo actually felt like a relief, like: 'Oh! Thank goodness! This is all actually fine because none of it is real.'

CAPRI SUN, CLEANING AND STRANGE CONVERSATIONS

My memories of the rest of the night are patchy. I remember phoning my dad, only to panic when I heard his voice, realising that I didn't know what on earth to say. How could I articulate what was going on? I think I managed, 'Something's happened. You need to get off the train', before handing the phone over to a police officer.

Two hours must have passed when the Air Ambulance doctor asked my mum and I to sit down at the kitchen table. I had an overwhelming sinking feeling, my palms were dripping with sweat, my heart started to race. I read what he was going to say through his body language and his facial expression: the half-smile he gave in an attempt to comfort us as he asked if we'd like a glass of water. He then sat down next to us, and was very straightforward, but not unkind, when he told us: 'At this point it's very unlikely that Sam will survive; if he does he will be severely brain damaged.' A sentence that literally took my breath away. He 'will' be severely brain damaged:

there was no 'might' or 'could' about it; it was simply a fact. My mum broke down and all I could do was stay calm, hug her and try my best to reassure her. I kept telling her how Sam had the best possible chance because these people were some of the best in the world at what they do. I repeated it over and over again: 'They are the best people in the world at this.' And they'd been such a long time in my house working on Sam – hours. They never gave up, just worked and worked and worked. Tried and tried and tried. They wouldn't have done that if there'd been no hope, would they?

A police officer sat with me for most of the night as well as a family friend, Ashley, who we'd called to come over while Mum went with the police to the hospital. I remember discussing who we should call, both of us saying what a cruel thing it was to do to someone – asking them to witness the trauma of what was going on but simultaneously wanting someone who we thought would be able to handle it.

The police officer who looked after me was called Jordan. He was a massive man. Ex-army and covered in tattoos. He looked like the sort of guy you definitely wouldn't cross. But appearances can be deceiving because he was incredibly kind to me and Tom. He showed me his tattoos, talking me through what they meant and where and why he'd got them. We also went through all the kit on his vest, him explaining what everything was for and how it worked. I was sipping on a Capri Sun, and it was around this time that my back started to feel very sore, and I couldn't stop shaking. Intermittently, I'd have to break the conversation to run off and throw up.

You could tell Jordan was affected by being there. It was obvious that everyone found the whole thing horrible. Another police officer took a statement from me, and I explained what I'd seen and what I'd done. He was really young – must only have been in his early or mid-twenties – and I remember he kept wincing and grimacing as I was talking, hiding his eyes behind his notepad to avoid looking at me.

At about 3 a.m., the police told me I should probably go to bed and try to get some rest. When I got up to my room, I remembered that I'd said I'd bring the example school hoodie into class the next day. (My school 'house' was called Allan and every year we'd make 'Allan Boys' hoodies to sell. I was meant to bring the example hoodie into school to show everyone.) I took it back downstairs and handed it to Ashley, whose son, Jonny, is a mate of mine from school, asking if he wouldn't mind passing it on. I could probably have been excused for not doing that, but at the time it seemed like quite a normal thing to worry about: 'Oh shit, how am I going to get the hoodie to school now?' Funny how our minds try to ground us in reality during times like these by focusing on the banal.

I went back upstairs, intending to get into bed, but curiosity led me into my parents' bedroom where the paramedics had moved Sam so they had more space. Seeing the state of that room was like running face-first into a brick wall. Medical debris was everywhere and there was a huge amount of blood on the carpet. I realised that I absolutely couldn't let my parents come home to that, so I started cleaning up: picking up syringe caps and all sorts of medical packaging from the floor and moving a rug to cover up the blood.

When describing the 'aftershock' of that night, I always catch myself saying, 'I woke up the next morning', when of course I didn't, because in order to wake up you must first fall asleep. So, it's more correct to say: when I stumbled out of bed the next morning, I found my mum, dad and our GP in the living room. They told me that Sam hadn't made it. I didn't really react to the news, I guess because it was as if they were telling me something I already knew.

Sitting there, the silence was deafening, broken only occasionally by the sound of sobs. There's a phrase people often use to describe the aftermath of trauma: 'it was like a bomb had gone off'. And there really is no better comparison. Time had stopped and everything was in pieces. You don't know what to do with yourself; you don't know which way is up or down. And it's all just so *enormous*.

My dad told us: 'It'll be okay, we'll get through this as a family', but my immediate and visceral response was not one of comfort, but anger. It descended like a red mist. How could Sam have been so cruel to have done this to us? How could he have been so *selfish*? But, as quickly as those thoughts arrived, they were crushed by this overwhelming and weirdly continuous feeling of emotional nothingness. The single most prevalent emotion I felt was: nothing. I just wanted to be left alone and not have to be around anything or anyone. Not have to see other people and respond to their numbness, their horror, their grief, their shock. Not to have to think about how my face must look exactly like theirs and then remember anew, every single time, why. Not to have to see the police walking in and out of the house, making it feel like somewhere else. Not to have to witness the physical wreckage of the night before, all of which was just more proof that it was real.

I had to get out, I had to escape.

MENTAL WHACK-A-MOLE

The morning of 22 January 2018, I took Tippy, our dog, out for a walk. And I walked and walked and walked, with no idea where I was going. I wailed and cried. But then, for the next mile, I felt nothing – and that numbness was such a relief, because soon the pain would come again. At some point, I found myself sitting at the edge of some woods. It had turned into a beautiful January morning – blue skies and unseasonably warm. The irony, huh? (Is that irony? I don't know, but you get what I mean.) I sat back against a tree, physically and emotionally wracked with exhaustion and shock. The constant rollercoaster of feeling nothing . . . and then falling into a pit of emotion and doubling over with an excruciating pain that felt like a stabbing sensation. And then my brain would switch into firefighting mode and smother the pain, stopping the flames spreading. It was like playing a game of mental whack-a-mole.

I decided to send Sam a text. (I want to say here that I'm sharing this message to show where my mind was at the time. I wouldn't send it now. I know more now. But I think it's important to understand the conflict of emotions and how they can manifest – all in one moment, all in one message. I'll reiterate that suicide is not a choice, and therefore cannot be something that is someone's fault. If you're feeling suicidal, the last thing you need is to feel guilty about how you're feeling.)

It's not like you can read this but for some reason it feels like you can. Why Sam? You have no idea how much pain you've caused everyone. It's horrific. I tried to save you, I spent half an hour doing CPR on you. That image will haunt me for the rest of my life. Now I'm not blaming you for causing this pain because this wasn't you. You were a fun joking boy who everyone loved. And over the last few months someone else has taken his place. I don't know that person but whoever that was has ripped our lives apart. You will be remembered forever and mourned by so many. We all love you Sam. More than you ever realised. I miss you so much. I'm crying writing this message. You have no idea how much you mean to so many people. I will never forget you and will always love you. Ben

And then, while I was sitting against this tree, looking out over a ploughed cornfield and the seemingly endless rolling hills of the Kent countryside, a plane flew over. Seeing this plane triggered one of the most profound and unexplainable feelings I've ever had. Everything in my life had stopped, had shattered, and I was in emotional vertigo, but as I watched that plane fly across the sky I realised that fuck all had actually changed for the rest of the world.

I could hear cars in the distance, people travelling to wherever they were going, absolutely unaware that anything was amiss. The birds in the trees were still singing, people were still going about their daily business, and hell, right at that exact moment Tippy took a shit in front of me. I'm not kidding and I'm sorry for being gross, but it's totally true. She even turned her head and stared at me sheepishly while she did it, as if she were saying, 'Sorry I couldn't help it.' And I started laughing because it was so ridiculous.

Everyone thinks they know – or that they have an idea – how they'll feel if something terrible like this happens to them. We like to believe that we understand emotions. But I don't think we have the faintest clue in reality. Because, sitting in those woods, with my life in pieces, having just experienced a level of trauma that will haunt me for the rest of my life, I was suddenly hit with a sense of ... peacefulness. In a distorted way, realising that the world was just continuing as normal – that birds were singing, cars were driving, planes were flying and Tippy was shitting – made me feel entirely present in the moment, possibly for the very first time in my life. I wasn't thinking, I was just feeling. I was just *there*. And that gave me a sense of peace.

WHY THESE STORIES MATTER

The trauma of suicide sends shockwaves through families and communities. In Sam's case, literally thousands of people were affected. Every suicide is a ripple that turns into a wave that sweeps through so many lives. The trauma is in the empty seat in class on Monday; it's in the tears in the police officer's eyes; it's in the hugs the paramedics give their families at the end of their shifts; and it's in a 999 call handler's memory of a panicked kid laugh-crying hysterically down the phone as he gives his brother CPR.

But Sam's death wasn't a one-off that year. He was one of over six and a half thousand people to take their own lives in the UK in 2018.[1] It's easy to become numb to statistics – especially when the figures get so big – and everyone's eyes glaze over and the truth of what they mean gets lost. So I made a graphic representing everyone who died by suicide the same year that Sam did.

Thank you for reading my story. Thank you for being open to understanding the trauma, the grief, and the loss caused by just one of the figures in the graphic on the opposite page. If you care about my tale, then you care about every single one of those figures represented. Look again at that image and tell me it's okay. The devastation that suicide brings affects hundreds of thousands of people every single year, and it will continue to do so until we make preventing it a priority.

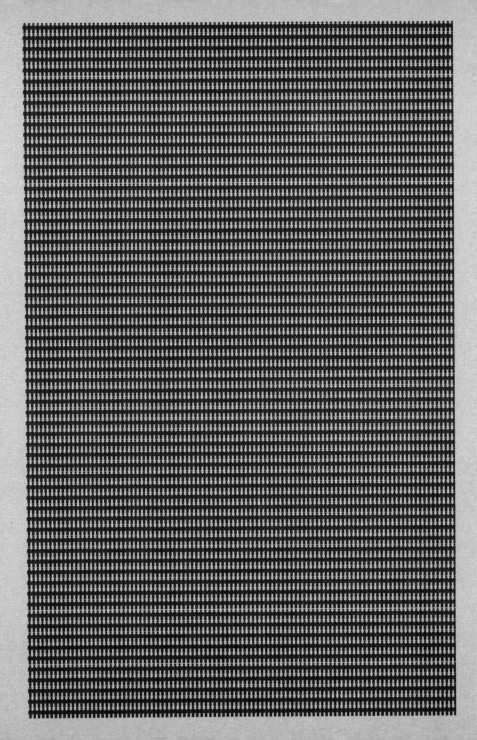

HOW TO DO CPR

That I knew what to do when I opened the door to Sam's bedroom has saved me a lot of additional pain. The fact that I was able to try to help Sam immediately not only brought the situation under control but was invaluable in giving Sam the best possible chance of survival. I've often said that I was thankful to be given the opportunity to perform CPR on Sam. Yes, it was traumatic, but it allowed me to have one final, loving moment with him. It was the last time I touched him, the last time I spoke to him, the last time I saw him. And, being in a position of trying to save his life, well, in a weird way I've found that very settling. The paramedics told me I'd done really well and everything I possibly could have, and I have found deep comfort in those words.

Finding someone unconscious and not breathing is thankfully very rare, but it is incredibly important that if it does ever happen to you (fingers crossed it won't), you know what to do. If someone is having a cardiac arrest (i.e. their heart has stopped) they will die if they don't receive immediate medical help. Knowing what to do means you'll not only be in a position to save someone's life, but it'll make you feel better within the moment and afterwards. Regardless of the outcome, you'll know you did all you could. These instructions are from the British Heart Foundation[2] and I hope you'll read them and perhaps practise. Better yet, speak to your school or workplace about putting on a first aid session. That we don't all get taught this as a matter of course is mad.

STEP 1: SHAKE AND SHOUT

* If you come across someone who is unconscious, always check for danger and look for risks before you start helping.
* Someone in cardiac arrest either won't be breathing at all or won't be breathing normally and will be unconscious (i.e. unresponsive). ('Unconscious' is actually a vague term – consciousness is more on a spectrum than a simple yes or no. In this instance it means the person isn't alert or responsive. They can't tell you what happened or where they are, they won't respond to your voice and they also won't respond to pain. Detailing their level of responsiveness, rather than saying that they're 'unconscious', will enable the professionals to better help the patient once they arrive.) You can check their level of responsiveness by shaking them gently.
* Shout for help. If someone is nearby, ask them to stay as you might need them. If you are alone, shout loudly to attract attention, but don't leave the patient.

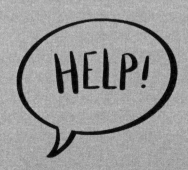

»

STEP 2: CALL EMERGENCY SERVICES

✳ If the person is not breathing or not breathing normally: ask someone to call the emergency services immediately and ask for an ambulance; also, ask someone for a public access defibrillator (PAD). If there's no one around, make the call yourself before starting compressions.

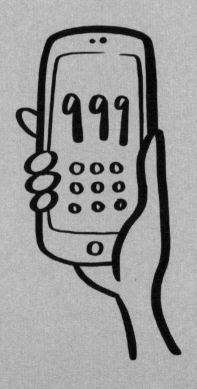

STEP 3: COVER MOUTH AND NOSE WITH CLOTH

* If you think there's a risk of infection, lay a towel or a piece of clothing over the mouth and nose. Don't put your face close to theirs. If you're sure the person is breathing normally, then put them in the recovery position.

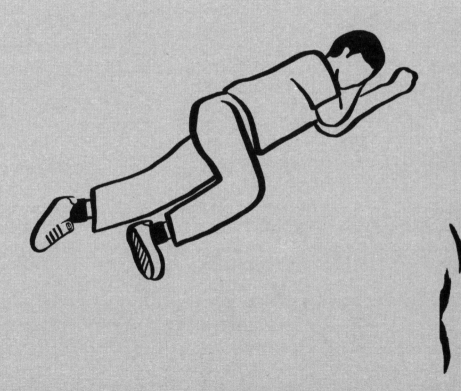

»

STEP 4: GIVE CHEST COMPRESSIONS

* Do not give rescue breaths at this time. Kneel next to the person.
* Place the heel of one hand in the centre of their chest. Place your other hand on top of the first. Interlock your fingers.
* With straight arms, use the heel of your hand to push the breastbone down firmly and smoothly, so that the chest is pressed down between 5 and 6 cm, and release. Do this at a rate of 100 to 120 chest compressions per minute – that's around two per second.

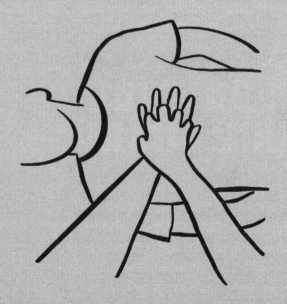

STEP 5: KEEP GOING

* Keep going until professional help arrives and takes over, or the person starts to show signs of regaining consciousness, such as coughing, opening their eyes, speaking, or breathing normally. If you're feeling tired, and there's someone nearby to help, instruct them to continue.

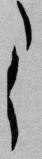

»

WHAT TO DO IF YOU/SOMEONE ELSE IS GOING INTO SHOCK

Another important thing to be able to deal with is shock. Shock is a medical emergency and is a life-threatening condition. It's brought on by the sudden drop in blood flow around the body. It may be the result of trauma, heatstroke, blood loss, an allergic reaction, poisoning, severe burns or an infection, among other causes.

Signs of shock are:

* clammy skin
* pale skin
* blue tinge to lips or fingernails
* rapid pulse
* rapid breathing
* nausea or vomiting
* enlarged pupils
* weakness or fatigue
* dizziness or fainting
* changes in mental state like confusion, agitation or anxiousness.

If you suspect someone is in shock, call the emergency services and then immediately:

* Lay the person down and elevate their legs and feet above the height of their heart. Don't do this, however, if it is going to cause them further injury or pain.
* If the person becomes unconscious, unresponsive and stops breathing, begin CPR.
* Loosen tight clothing and, if cold, cover them with a blanket.
* Don't let the person eat or drink anything.
* If you suspect the person is having an allergic reaction and you have access to an epinephrine injector (EpiPen) then administer as described on its instructions.
* If the person is bleeding, hold pressure on the bleeding area using a towel or sheet.
* If the person vomits or begins bleeding from the mouth, and there isn't a spinal injury suspected, turn them on their side to prevent choking.

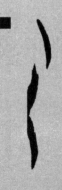

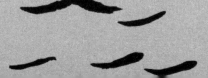

TAKEAWAYS

- Trauma affects everyone in different ways. There's no 'correct' way to behave during a traumatic event, so don't judge yourself or others for acting out of character, for going into shock, for freezing or for behaving in ways that may seem strange (i.e. by laughing).

- Learning CPR and basic first aid is a brilliant way of ensuring you'll be in the best possible position to help someone should the need ever arise. It won't only possibly save a life, but will also help you to feel better about having done all you could.

- Thank you for reading this chapter. It means a lot to me. It's important to understand as much as possible about suicide and suicide prevention in order to help.

CHAPTER 3

WTF JUST HAPPENED?

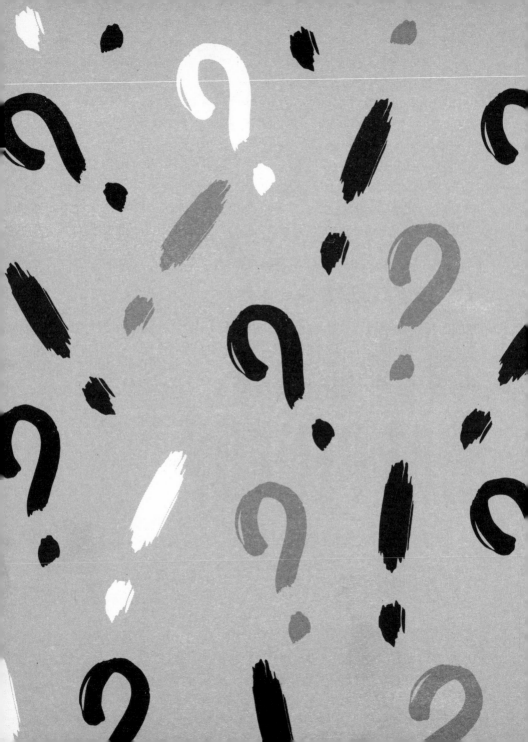

Returning back from that walk in the woods was horrendous. My house was suddenly 'the place where it had happened' and it felt suffocating. My mind was all over the place, I wasn't thinking straight at all. I wanted so desperately for everything to be normal again, and on a normal Monday I'd have been at school – so that's exactly where I decided I should be.

I usually did army cadet training on Monday afternoons at school. I loved being part of the army cadets – so much so, in fact, that I was actually Colour Sergeant West. How fancy is that? Much of the personal growth I experienced at secondary school – i.e. me turning from a green banana into a yellow one – can be directly attributed to my time in the cadets. Over five years, I'd worked my way up to leader of our school contingent. People wouldn't believe it now (actually, anyone who's seen some of my Instagram videos might . . .), but I really enjoyed barking orders and marching around! That day, I figured that maybe if I acted like nothing had changed, nothing would have changed. Maybe if I ignored reality, it wouldn't be reality. Maybe the world would realise it had made a mistake.

I'd already convinced myself that this was a fantastic idea when, as I was leaving the house, some family friends arrived. I loved them dearly, but I absolutely couldn't deal with that. I couldn't face other people's sympathy, pity or horror. There's also the very British thing of still feeling as though you have to 'look after' guests even when you're dealing with the shittiest situation on the planet. In the midst of complete carnage, when you're standing in the rubble of what used to be your life, you'll still offer to make people a cup of tea, ask how they are and apologise for the stale Digestives. And, at that precise moment, I wanted nothing to do with it.

So off I went to school.

Everyone at Cranbrook Grammar had been told about Sam. I remember my mum saying she'd have to call the school ... and then wondering what on earth to say. How do you even start to explain it? But she must have found some words, because they knew, and the news hit the place like a wrecking ball. The analogy 'it was like a bomb had gone off' came up a lot again, students recalling how the shock turned them into zombies, staggering through a suddenly unfamiliar land-scape. Many were told they could go home if they wanted.

So school was already a strange place for everyone that day ... and then I turned up. My brain had gone so far into overdrive trying to fabricate some sort of normality that I practically *skipped* into the grounds. When I saw some people I knew, I went over and said, in a jolly way: 'Hey! How's every-one doing?' I mean, what on earth must they have thought?! I was laughing and smiling while everyone looked at me like I'd sailed in on a flying carpet. You could see the ques-tions on their faces. Had the school got it wrong? Was Sam actually okay? Was this all some really shitty elaborate joke?

It wasn't long before a teacher pulled me to one side and I remember being really surprised by how serious he was. I had genuinely tricked myself into believing that it had all been an awful dream. A nightmare I could forget at cadets because I'd always felt safe there and, best of all, in control. I called the shots – quite literally – so heading there seemed like an obvious plan. At least I would know what I was doing. And so, less than 24 hours after finding Sam, I was standing in front of a group of students talking them through weapons handling. Everyone was staring at me in a glazed-over way. It was the look you'd give someone who'd turned an unnatural colour; an uncomfortable, 'Is this guy okay and is what he's got contagious?' stare. I didn't care though, because for the first time all day I felt like I'd got a handle back on my life. (And, as it turns out, the cadets would continue to be an escape for me over the coming months.)

But inevitably the mirage faded and reality punched me in the face. All at once, I suddenly, desperately wanted to go home. The switch had been flicked and I sagged with exhaustion. So, as randomly as I arrived, I left again and, on the way to my car, two people from my year group stopped and hugged me. I didn't know them too well but that hug was much needed. I thanked them, opened my car door, got in and immediately broke down. (*I* broke down, not the car. What incredibly shitty luck would it have been for my car to choose that moment to break down?) I sat in the school car park and sobbed and sobbed, hitting the steering wheel so hard I made the horn go off. Control, it seemed, was firmly out of my hands again.

MASKS ARE MANDATORY

I arrived home to a stale, strange atmosphere. The police, doctors, neighbours and friends had all left, leaving just me, Tom, Mum and Dad. This was the first time it had been our family group without Sam. Well, just us and dozens of bunches of flowers. And so much food! People were dropping off dishes of food and flowers on the doorstep and quickly leaving, not wanting to intrude. The gesture was kind, compassionate and beautiful, but it was also a visual and aural reminder of what had happened – the house looked and smelled different now.

That night, we sat around the dinner table and I remember cracking a joke about how cruel it was to send a hay-fever sufferer flowers. Like, wasn't I crying enough?! You don't see me sending someone allergic to bees a beehive when they're upset. The joke got a few tepid smiles as we pushed the food around on our plates. None of us felt like eating. Or talking. Or catching each other's eyes. I managed a few mouthfuls but couldn't stomach anything more. And, it's not like I wasn't hungry either – I was, in the same way that I was *so tired* but couldn't sleep. Sam's absence around the table was obviously glaring, but I was so shocked, tired and withdrawn it didn't hit me properly right then.

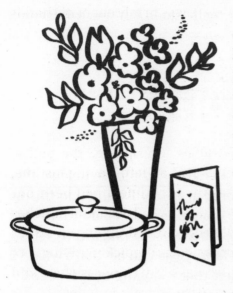

After dinner (if you can call it that) I decided to brave looking at my phone. Oh, my phone! Where do I start in discussing what a blessing and a curse that thing is? I'd deliberately ignored it for most of the day. I knew what was happening with it: the messages and missed calls from friends and family piling in. And, as much as that support was incredible, it was too *real* and over-whelming. Also, you feel this obligation to respond and I had no idea what to say. But I knew I'd have to face it sometime, so I dove in, checking Facebook, Instagram and Snapchat, and every message I opened brought the pain right back to the surface. 'I'm so sorry to hear about Sam; anything I can do to help just let me know' – that sentiment was echoed *hundreds* of times. People also shared fond memories of Sam and offered to go for walks or have talks. One person even sent loads of photos of her dogs, which was a welcome relief. I tried to reply to all of them. It was difficult because, as upsetting as the messages were to read, they were also really comforting. I genuinely appreciated them and so wanted to say thank you for the sentiment.

One of the messages that really stood out was a voicemail from PC Jordan, the policeman who had looked after me the night before. He said:

> 'I'm so sorry about what's happened, mate. Look after yourself and the family and if there's anything you need or anything I can do to help just call.'

What a legend. And he was right – I did have to look after myself. I wanted to stay strong at home, I wanted to lift the mood. I've always been like that: a rescuer. I'll do whatever I can to make other people feel better, so if that means telling jokes to a recently bereaved family you can bet that's what I'll do. (What do you call a hen that's looking at a lettuce? A chicken sees a salad. I'll see myself out . . .)

One of my biggest coping mechanisms is laughing; laughing can make everything seem good again for a fraction of a moment. So, equipped with my admittedly *very* shit jokes, there I was trying to give people that moment of relief when actually I really needed to cry my heart out to someone who would just let me. My default response of trying to have a laugh and make light of things is a classic avoidance technique. I remember people saying they were worried I wasn't 'processing' what had happened because I kept trying to deflect from it, but I wasn't in any fit state to start processing. Laughter was my mask and I needed it.

There are famous cases of people 'not appearing shocked or sad enough' after a personal tragedy (for example, Gerry and

Kate McCann were put under the microscope for years for not 'doing grief properly'). But the truth is, there is no 'correct' way of grieving or dealing with trauma. Putting on a mask and pretending to be okay is much easier than weeping in front of a bunch of strangers. I've spoken with my mum about this since and she admitted that, as a mother, she questioned how Kate McCann had remained so seemingly emotionless in press interviews and on TV – but now she understands exactly how and why she did: numbness, protection, stoicism, shock, anger, frustration, fear. The list goes on.

On which note, I want you to do something for me right now please: put on a massive smile, letting your face light up. Maybe even let out a small chuckle. Make sure the smile reaches your eyes. Comes pretty easy, right? It's sometimes much easier to do that than it is to break down and expose your raw emotions and then deal with people's expectations, judgements, awkwardness or 20 questions.

But the mask always slips, of course. And, as much as I'd have liked to be able to keep it on for ever, that first evening it dropped. In my self-appointed role as 'rescuer', I knew I didn't want to let my family see, so I went out and met up with a good friend of mine; we sat in my car, I rested my head on her shoulder and sobbed. She let me sound off to her and simply listened. I was, and still am, very grateful for that.

Another time I remember my mask slipping and having to quickly pull it back on was a few days later, when we went out for breakfast as a family at a nearby truckers' cafe. I went to get cutlery for everyone and returned to the table with five sets. I put them down, quickly realised and then took one set back. That gave me such a lump in my throat. But because I didn't want to upset anyone else by being upset myself, I didn't say anything and buried the feelings.

But they couldn't and wouldn't stay buried all the time, and over the next few weeks and months that feeling would hit me whenever I was alone. I'd sweat, shake and feel sick in bed, my mind racing, churning and spinning. I'd look at the clock and realise another night had passed with no sleep. I could pretend as much as I liked that I was handling shit and being stoical in front of other people, but I couldn't outrun the emotional fog when I was by myself. And the fact that I could put on a mask so successfully when I was with others made me question myself. When you've been through a hideous and bizarre experience, you have no idea how you'll react (especially when in public), and analysing and judging your emotions and behaviour is pointless and damaging.

So, of course, that's exactly what I did.

ONE TICKET FOR THE GUILT AND SHAME ROLLERCOASTER PLEASE

'Sam left thinking I didn't care,' I wrote to myself on the back of a piece of paper soon after he died. 'He thought I wouldn't be affected by his death because I didn't love him. That hurts.

Now I want to prove him wrong. Not that he will ever know he was. Maybe instead I'm trying to prove it to myself. I need to prove to myself that I did care. Fuck, I miss him.'

The emotions that hit me the hardest, and that hurt the most, were undoubtedly guilt and shame. As the days went by, and as I thought about it more and more, I became convinced that Sam's death was my fault. During dinner that night, on the 21 January, he and I had an argument. He stormed off upstairs and, as he was leaving, I said something under my breath that would haunt me for years. I really struggle to find a way to say this – it's something I've tried to keep buried and, previous to writing this book, I've never told anyone – but the last thing I ever said to Sam was, 'Fuck off'.

When I remembered that, it seemed to me that everything that had happened that night was my fault and I felt like I was drowning. My whole body tensed up, my chest felt like it was being squeezed in a vice, my heart started pounding hard, and I couldn't breathe.

Oh my God. This was all my fault.

Even when I tried to rationalise it, I was dragged back under by those two words. I felt like I had killed Sam. Imagine how you would feel if you found out that you'd actually killed someone. The horror of it. I couldn't believe what I'd done – I couldn't believe that I was the kind of person who would do that. The fear and guilt consumed me, ate me up, and quickly induced a deep sense of shame.

I want to clarify that I know *now* that what happened wasn't my fault. I realise that suicide isn't a choice, it's a symptom.

But it's taken me years to get to that point; to stop torturing myself with things I shoulda, coulda, or woulda done differently. In reality, Sam probably didn't even hear me. And, even if he had, it wouldn't have made any difference because that's not how depression and suicide work. Depression is an illness that can bubble away for years, and an off-the-cuff statement isn't going to cause someone's death.

But, at the time, I truly believed that I had killed my brother. And, worst of all, I couldn't tell anyone – none of my family or friends – because I was both deeply ashamed and honestly thought I might be arrested. It probably sounds like an overreaction, but I was genuinely petrified that I could go to prison.

GUILT AND SHAME IN A NUTSHELL

Guilt: a sense that you have done something wrong.
Shame: a sense that you yourself *are* wrong – that you are flawed as a person.

'Healthy' guilt is when the feeling's entirely justified (i.e. when you have actually done something wrong) and it prompts you to try to make amends or change your behaviour. The reason you feel guilty is because you recognise that what you did or what you're doing (or what you're *not* doing) goes against your values and so makes you uncomfortable. However, guilt can also be 'unhealthy': when you haven't actually done anything wrong. Unhealthy guilt can be caused by misunderstandings, self-doubt, low self-esteem, or societal and cultural expectations.

An example of healthy guilt might be when you cheated on an exam and feel that you have wronged other students and yourself. An example of unhealthy guilt is feeling bad for spending Sunday watching your favourite boxset in your pyjamas even though you have absolutely nothing else to do and aren't hurting anyone. You feel guilty because of some misplaced sense that you should be constantly 'doing'.

Both healthy and unhealthy guilt can lead to shame when your actions (or the way you perceive your actions) make you question whether or not you're a good or worthy person (i.e. 'What kind of

»

person would do something like that?'). Feelings of shame can also be entirely unrelated to any 'event' or circumstance, instead prompted by a belief that you're just 'wrong' inside – that you're in some way defective, not up to scratch or flawed. In order to try to run from or mask any of these feelings, you might indulge in damaging behaviours such as alcoholism, eating disorders, drug-taking, truancy or violence. What fun and games, eh?

People speak about guilt and shame a lot and often use the terms interchangeably when they're actually different. Recognising this difference is important, so you can understand what you're experiencing and how you can then best work through it (please see box on page 97). Guilt is what hit me first: 'I hurt Sam and because of that I've hurt everyone else too.' This then led to shame as I believed that what I'd done (what I *thought* I'd done) made me a bad person: 'Who would do something like that? What does that say about me? I must be a terrible human being.' Feeling such shame *really* hurt. It gave me such a low opinion of myself and shattered my self-esteem. I won't lie to you, at times that shame made me hate myself; I deeply hated who I thought I was. And I couldn't let on about any of it because I thought I'd done something that was not only morally reprehensible, but that might have landed me in trouble with the law, which was the last thing my family needed.

My guilt was definitely unhealthy – I hadn't actually done anything to Sam. We'd had a row. The kind of row all brothers have, every single day. The kind of row that, at any other time, would have been forgotten immediately. But my mind, injured by trauma and drowning in grief, became intoxicated with the idea that I'd caused this. It was something I understood: if I'd just done something differently, I could have prevented what happened. Believe it or not, that was a better thought at the time than the fact that suicide is a symptom of an illness that I didn't understand and had absolutely zero control over.

FOR LONG PERIODS, I'D FEEL ... NOTHING. AND THAT FUELLED MY SHAME. HOW COULD I NOT FEEL *ANYTHING?*

Another of the most common feelings I experienced at that time was complete numbness. The absence of any emotion whatsoever. For long periods, I'd feel ... nothing. And that fuelled my shame. How could I not feel *anything*? What was wrong with me? And the answer my exhausted brain came up with was obvious: I didn't love him. The numbness convinced me that I wasn't actually affected by Sam's death. That my ability to go to school the day after and crack jokes and muck about – to be normal – confirmed that there was something intrinsically wrong with me as a person. I was his older brother; why wasn't I there for him? Why didn't he feel comfortable talking to me? Why didn't I talk to him about it? The questions, the accusations, the numbness, the guilt, the shame – they were all unbearable.

And I couldn't tell a single person about any of this because I didn't want other people to feel the same way about me as I did about myself.

SLIDING DOORS

My various masks did a great job of convincing many people that I wasn't stuck in an emotional washing machine. There was the joker mask, the rescuer mask – and the busy mask. Hell, I could even kid myself occasionally that I was doing okay by keeping busy. A couple of days after Sam died, I emailed my A-Level teachers asking for work. That still makes me laugh looking back on it: I *hated* schoolwork, and there I was, asking for exam papers and lesson notes. Who was I?! What a contrast to the green banana who shouldn't sit any exams! But I'd have much rather studied the biology of plants than mope around feeling sad. (On which note though, has anyone ever opted to study biology because they're interested in plants?! I don't care how sugar goes up the xylem, or how a plant cell wall works – surely no one has ever found that remotely interesting? No offence to my biology teacher, who was great, but plant biology? Snore.)

School became an escape for me, both the work and the social side. My friends were incredible and I know how lucky I was to have such a supportive network at that time. For example, I wasn't really eating much at all, and one day, without making a big deal out of it, a group of mates told me we were all bunking off that afternoon to go to Wagamama's for lunch. I'm still not sure how they'd known it would help, but holy fucking moley that was the nicest meal I have had or will ever eat. I had ramen and gyozas. I ate all of it and, for the first time since Sam had died, I wasn't hungry. I felt more ener-gised, more upbeat, and like I was taking back control of the situation. It was such a relief.

That was a good moment. And there were a few. Pinpricks of light in a canvas of grief.

One very strange reaction I had, which to this day I find difficult to explain, was an overwhelming and irrational fear of closed doors. Doors to rooms, yes, but also cupboard doors and drawers. The idea of not knowing what was on the other side made me feel panicked. I would stand in front of a closed door and feel an actual physical fear. My heart would start racing, my palms would get sweaty and I would often have to walk away, waiting for my body to calm down before returning to try again.

I ended up telling my mum about it because I was getting concerned (and because it was seriously inconvenient) and we went to my GP. I described the feeling as akin to when you're watching a horror movie and are anticipating a jump scare. Or like when you hear a noise downstairs in the middle of the night and you're on your own. It's that pre-emptive expectation that heightens your senses and brings on a feeling of anxiety. But rather than experiencing that when faced with the Candyman or a burglar, I was drenched in sweat contemplating my bloody sock drawer. I know some instinctual part of my subconscious or psyche was imagining Sam on the other side of those doors.

The doctor prescribed me anti-anxiety medication. (The subject of mental health and medication is a complicated one and not something I'm going to dive into. I'm not an expert and it's not what this book is about. From my point of view, it's important that people are given access, options and information, so they can make a personal choice – my main worry being that people don't know there are options or can't access them.) For me personally, I found it reassuring to have the pills rather than feeling I needed to take them. It was more a case of knowing that if I felt particularly anxious one day, they were there. And they're still there, sitting on my chest of drawers, because I ended up only taking one (don't worry, I know meds expire). My extreme reactions to doors thankfully passed relatively quickly and within a week or two my mind accepted that my sock drawer was full of nothing but socks and maybe a few old pennies.

I soon discovered that 'irrational anxiety' was a symptom of post-traumatic stress and that everyone was concerned about me developing post-traumatic stress disorder (PTSD – please see box on page 108). That definitely sounded like something I should try to ward off if at all possible, so when it was suggested that I see a counsellor some time later, I said yes.

Now, I had no idea what to expect from counselling except what I'd seen on TV: stern-looking therapists doodling on a pad while their patients lie on a couch staring at the ceiling revealing their deepest darkest secrets. I was tentative about experiencing that first-hand, but was really looking forward to lying on one of those fancy half-couches. Imagine my disappointment then when I turned up to my first appointment and was offered a boring chair to sit on. The counsellor, a pleasant, slight man we'll call Fred, invited me to start talking and I did, even though I found the whole thing quite uncomfortable (not the chair, which was actually fine; more the general vibe). I couldn't help thinking that I was simply repeating my police statement and wondering what on earth the point of that was? And then things took a quite spectacular turn.

Fred told me that he'd asked his father (who we'll call Philip) whether he should take me on as a new client. So far, so strange (what professional counsellor runs potential patients past their dad first?) but then came the big reveal. It turns out – and I'll say this as bluntly as Fred himself did – that his dad was dead. Fred told me how he'd been discussing me and my situation with his dead father and it was his dad who'd convinced him that he could help me (cheers, Phil. RIP). He then starts *crying* about it. Both about my situation and his dad's response. *This man is not okay*, I'm thinking while wondering where to look. It felt very much like I had become the counsellor, asking about his dad and dishing out condolences, while Fred reached for the tissues to dry his eyes. *Were those meant for him or me?* I thought.

Safe to say, I didn't go back. While he was a very nice person and I'm sure some people would get on with him really well, I left that place and laughed the entire way home. I couldn't believe what I'd just witnessed! So thank you, Fred, for your time, and thank you, Philip, for your hilariously unexpected involvement.

I did end up finding a counsellor that I clicked with much better in 2020 and I credit the work we did together for helping to get me where I am today. It's really important to know that not every counsellor or every kind of therapy will be right for you. There can be an expectation that because they're the expert, you should put up and shut up, but they're just people at the end of the day, and you'll feel more comfortable with some than with others. You have to find someone you get on with, who you trust, and whose specialisms work for you. Without trying to be sensationalist, if it goes well, your counsellor will likely know more about you than anyone else in your life. To be able to talk *that* candidly with someone takes a connection that can't be willed or forced. It can take time and involve a bit of trial and error. Please don't give up and don't let a bad experience put you off for good. Again, I wish I'd been told this earlier because my time with Fred really did make me think the whole thing was completely batshit. Luckily, I gave it another go and it was a game changer.

WHAT IS 'GRIEF'?

Grief is an emotional reaction to the loss of someone or something that's important to you. Every single one of us will be exposed to death during our lifetime and so will experience grief. People mainly associate it with sadness, but there's an abundance of feelings you may or may not experience during bereavement. I'll be honest – it's shit. The fact you can't anticipate how you're going to feel one minute to the next isn't fun and you'll definitely find yourself questioning the process – but there is no right or wrong way to grieve, just as there's no definitive timeline to it.

Common stages of grief are:

Denial: 'This isn't happening.' It's common to initially react to loss with sensations of numbness and shock. It's your body's way of temporarily dealing with the rush of overwhelming emotions and sensations.

Anger: You may feel frustrated and helpless and those feelings can turn to anger – anger at the world, at the people around you or at the person who's died.

Bargaining: This is the 'what if . . .' or the 'if only . . .' stage when you question why it happened and what you or someone else could have done differently.

Depression: A feeling of intense sadness and loss. You may cry a lot, feel vulnerable, not be able to sleep or eat, experience regret or loneliness, and a whole host of other really fun emotions.

Acceptance: When you accept the reality of what has happened and start processing what it means. Acceptance doesn't mean you don't care any more, it simply means that you understand it can't be changed.

These stages aren't linear or chronological. You can flit between them, back and forth, up and down, side to side, left foot, right foot, do the hokey-cokey and turn around. Grief, by its very nature, is a messy and complicated business. But the fact it's messy IS ENTIRELY NORMAL. I'm shouting that because I wish someone had explained it to me.

»

WHAT IS PTSD?

Post-Traumatic Stress Disorder (PTSD) is a mental health condition, specifically an anxiety disorder, brought about by highly stressful, frightening and distressing events. PTSD is often associated with soldiers – in the First World War the term 'shell shocked' was coined to describe soldiers suffering with PTSD, and it's still something that affects the armed forces today (a 2019 study found that PTSD risk increased by 170 per cent for UK service personnel deployed to Iraq and/or Afghanistan[1]). But you don't have to be a soldier or have been involved in a war to develop the disorder – any exposure to traumatic events can increase the risk.

If you experience something traumatic, such as a road accident, assault, robbery, abuse or serious health problems, you'll most likely experience post-traumatic stress (PTS).[2] PTS is an entirely normal and natural response to being exposed to highly stressful situations and you'll experience both physical and mental heightened anxiety. After a period of time, this will fade. However, if it doesn't fade and you remain in a heightened physical and mental state for over a month – reliving the experience over and over again – and if your usual de-stressing coping mechanisms aren't working, you may have PTSD. And, to add another complication into the mix, the symptoms may not start immediately after the experience, but months or sometimes even years afterwards.[3]

Treatment for PTSD is available in the form of talking therapies and medication. The sooner help is sought, the better the chances are of recovery. (Chronic PTSD will need to be treated on a more long-term basis.) If you think you may be experiencing either PTS or PTSD, please speak to your doctor.

FIRST STEPS TO GETTING THERAPY

I make the analogy that finding appropriate therapy is a bit like going to a car wash – you're faced with dozens of options that effectively all offer the same thing, leaving you thinking, 'What's the difference between Economy, Bronze, Platinum and Platinum+ service? I just want to wash my car.' There isn't a one-size-fits-all with therapy either – there are dozens of different types. For example, CBT (Cognitive Behavioural Therapy), humanist, group, art, play, integrative, psychodynamic and so on. If one doesn't work for you, that doesn't mean there's a problem with you, with therapy in general, or with the therapist. If one type of car wash doesn't do a good job, it doesn't mean your car is never going to be clean.

To start investigating your options:

You can go to your GP, who can make a referral to NHS support (if your case fits certain criteria). (Doctors in hospitals can also make referrals.)

》

You can self-refer to some NHS support services, including drug and alcohol services and IAPT (a branch of the NHS mental health service that provides talking therapies). Please visit https://www.nhs.uk/mental-health/nhs-voluntary-charity-services/nhs-services/how-to-access-mental-health-services/ to find out more.

As already mentioned, there are issues with the public system. It is complicated, confusing and stretched very thin. There also appears to be a severe lack of communication between the NHS and the charity sector, to everyone's detriment. Some people are surprised to learn that many charities can offer free counselling to people with no waiting times.

If you search Hub of Hope (UK nationwide) you can find all private and charitable services in your area. Young Minds has also launched Bayo, a mental health wellbeing group specifically for the Black community, helping Black people to locate local services.

You can also pay for private counselling. Just please make sure the therapist and their practice is appropriately accredited by a recognised governing organisation. (Of course, the fact that people can pay to skip the queue raises its own issues.)

The above is obviously UK-specific, but charities and mental health organisations exist around the world. You can speak to your doctor, ask people you trust, try online forums or use a simple google search to find the support you need.

LOOKING BACK ON THAT TIME NOW

I want to put on my Mental Health Campaigner hat now and reiterate something: every year, tens of thousands of people go through what I had to go through and lose loved ones to suicide. I hope I've painted a picture that not only does justice to how absolutely awful that situation is, but also how terrible the following weeks and months can be. The truth of it is very simple: had I been a different person and had I not coped with this in the way that I did, there is a very real possibility that I could have developed quite severe mental illness myself as a result. Tragically, there's also a *very* real possibility that I too might have eventually taken my own life. Research has found that people bereaved by suicide are at a high risk of suicide themselves,[4] and, having read my story thus far, you can probably understand why that's the case.

It is a horrific thing to go through and the level of support offered to me was simply unacceptable. My parents were assigned a 'family liaison officer' via the police. However, said liaison officer handed them some leaflets and, to all intents and purposes, left us all to it. I wasn't spoken to one-on-one by anyone at all. The fact that no professional took me aside and said, 'This is what's going to happen next and you might feel like this' is unbelievable. Had they taken the time to speak to me – discussing counselling options (which didn't involve a therapist that communes with the dead *eye roll*) and explaining how guilt and shame are entirely natural responses to grief and trauma – I potentially could have avoided a lot of the trouble I found myself in.

It was as if my family were treated as part of a package grief deal, when that shouldn't have been the case. The World Health Organization (WHO) has identified that as well as implementing 'universal' suicide prevention strategies that target the general population, countries should also investigate and implement 'selective' prevention strategies that target specific at-risk groups.[5] My family's individual experiences of Sam and of his death were entirely different. I needed someone to recognise that, because when no one does you begin to wonder whether your responses are weird, strange, unusual, unexpected or shameful. If no one acknowledges that you might feel like shit, you wonder whether you actually should feel like shit or if the shit that you're feeling is the wrong kind.

We need robust, effective support systems in place to prop up families bereaved by sudden and violent death. The onus cannot be on the victim to reach out for support; it must be a proactive approach that checks on the welfare of those involved and clearly outlines the options available. Maybe support was offered to me, maybe I just don't remember being offered it, but I can say with certainty that no one ever called to check if I was okay following our initial involvement with the emergency services, and the way I look at it now, that's not good enough. Yes, I know there's a lot to be said here about budgets and staffing, yadda yadda yadda, but there are systems in place that aren't working, there is money being spent on the wrong things and there are small changes that could make huge differences. If we don't roll out proper, effective bereavement support we are failing at implementing the selective prevention that the WHO has stated is so important to the reduction of suicide.

MEMORIES AND MOTIVATION

At this point, our fridge was filled to bursting with food and our house filled to bursting with flowers. Sneezing through my Special K, I might as well have been eating breakfast in a flower meadow. People's generosity was really moving – so much so that we simply ran out of space for it all. We started thinking that there must be a better way for people to show that they care. My dad had the idea of starting a fundraiser with all the money going to mental health charities specialising in helping people in Sam's position. 'Great plan!' we all said. And then, 'Are you mad?' when he set the fundraising target at £10,000. We'll never get 10 grand, we scoffed. But how wrong we were! It took just eight days to smash that target – and the fund simply kept on growing, soon hitting £30,000. And I was particularly delighted: not only did we raise a boatload of cash for brilliant charities, but, minus the flowers, I was finally able to breathe again in my own house.

My school was incredible in the aftermath. It would have been easy for everyone there to try to brush the tragedy under the carpet in a misguided attempt to preserve the school's reputation, but the teachers, students and leadership did the exact opposite. Whatever we as a family thought best, they had our backs. And, as a family, we also recognised that it was important for everyone there to get closure too – so a memorial service was organised for the whole school in March. Many of Sam's teachers spoke about their memories of him and about their own struggles in dealing with what had happened. My parents also spoke, thanking everyone for their support and explaining the importance of the causes we were fundraising for. And I wrote a speech for that day. I wanted to talk about mental illness and how important it was that we started having these conversations.

Here's a snippet from my speech:

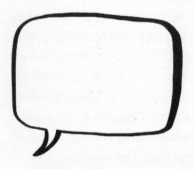

Normal: is it good enough? We've got so used to 'normal' that we have forgotten what that really means. We paint a glossy cover over a dark, twisted truth. Normal is hearing jokes about someone's appearance. Normal is mocking people that are different. Normal is laughing at people who aren't like you. Normal is belittling depression and mental illness. Normal is criticising people's every move. Normal is pushing others down to raise yourself up. Normal hurts people. I've been so desperate to get back to normal – but I don't want to rebuild that; I don't want to go back to that normal.

Mental illness can strike anyone. It doesn't matter who you are or what you've done, it can defeat the strongest soldiers. Don't try to fit in. Try to be the best version of yourself that you can be. Don't follow the crowds; grab life by the horns and live it to the best of your ability because if I've learned anything from this experience it's that life can be taken away in a heart-beat. Sam will be remembered for ever and mourned endlessly. I'll leave you with a quote: 'In the end, it's not the years in your life that counts, it's the life in your years.'

It was incredibly tough seeing first-hand the effect Sam's death had on the school, and particularly on his friends and year group – but the memorial had another immediate and extraordinary impact: the messages I received on social media started to change. The notes that I'd previously received saying things like, 'I hope you're doing okay' or 'I'm here if you want to talk', slowly changed to, 'I'm not doing okay' and 'I feel like I need to talk'. People started revealing their own struggles with mental illness, talking to me about their diagnoses of depression, anxiety or an eating disorder, or their worries about their friends and family. Some even revealed how they themselves had attempted suicide before.

It was beyond shocking to learn how many people were going through some really bad shit. I realised that nearly everyone around me was dealing with something that they didn't want anyone to know about. Just a few weeks ago I hadn't even known what mental illness was and now people I knew well, and also not at all, were revealing that it was a huge part of their lives. It had gone from a non-issue to something that had taken my brother's life and was affecting nearly everyone I knew. It was a realisation that shook me to the core. I desperately wanted to help everyone who was taking a chance by reaching out and telling me these things. Essentially, I wanted to stop what had happened to Sam from happening to anyone else. I certainly had my work cut out. I don't think I, or anyone else, could have predicted the impact those conversations would have on the trajectory of my life.

MESSAGES TO SEND TO SOMEONE EXPERIENCING LOSS

Here's a text I'd send to 17-year-old me:

'Hey mate, I heard about what happened. I'm so sorry, that must be awful for you. Genuinely, if you ever need someone to go for a walk with, to talk to or to make you a tea (I'll try and make it better than last time lol) then I would absolutely love to and all you need to do is let me know. We're all here for you. Sending lots of love x'

Remember:
* Don't overthink it. Better to send something than nothing at all.
* Ask yourself, what would I like to read or see?
* Don't be scared to be funny. If they'd enjoy a meme, send a meme.
* Don't expect a response. This isn't about you, it's about them. Don't take silence personally.
* Send a follow-up message in a week or month.
* If you're worried about them, tell them about SHOUT, a UK text-based support service, that they can message on 85258 for free. (See page 281 for other useful websites.)

TAKEAWAYS

- If someone you know is grieving, do reach out to them with a message of support or a picture of a cute dog. They may not answer, but they'll appreciate it. Also consider passing on the details of a text- or call-based support service, if one exists in your country. In the UK people can text SHOUT 85258 or call the Samaritans on 116 123 for free.

- Guilt and shame are normal reactions to trauma. Working out whether your guilt is healthy or unhealthy and whether it's contributing to a sense of shame can help in getting perspective on the situation.

- Grief is a natural emotional response to loss. It can be confusing and difficult (understatement of the decade) to navigate, but just knowing that can make the journey a bit easier. You are not weird for feeling like you're losing it.

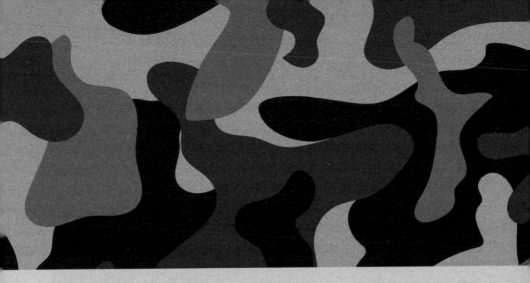

CHAPTER 4
WALK TO TALK

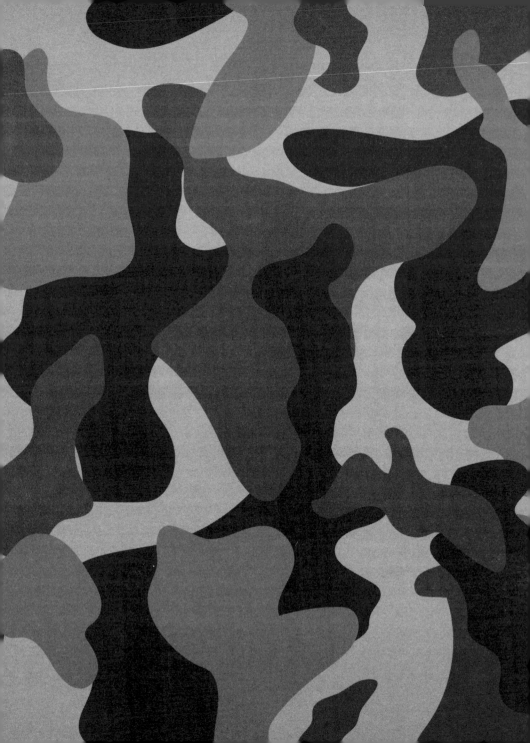

When you live in the middle of nowhere, walking fairly long distances becomes part of your daily life. For me and my friends, trudging for miles was not only necessary to get from A to B, but was also a key part of our cadet training and the expedition part of the Duke of Edinburgh's Award scheme (a youth awards activity programme, founded in the UK, that encourages life skills and community volunteering). And, while emotions weren't usually front and centre of our conversations, when my mates and I did finally get round to talking about stuff that mattered, it was often when we were lost in a cow field.

We clocked hundreds of miles on foot as kids, hiking through some really amazing places in amazing weather, and some really shit places in really shit weather. Our Duke of Edinburgh trip to Grey Hell, otherwise known as Dartmoor, sticks in my mind for being ruthlessly horrible: foggy, cold, wet, bleak and windy. But, the more awful it got, the more determined we were to successfully complete it. The communal discomfort really brought everyone closer together. We'd sing together through relentless downpours – 'Forever friends we will be!' (sorry, I'll stop there) – and learn way too much about each other (no, I don't want to know what you left behind in that hole in the ground, thanks). Weirdly, that trip also taught me how to prepare rice properly after my mate Seb didn't take too well to the dish I'd 'cooked' earlier. (I thought you just had to bring rice to the boil. I didn't know there was simmering involved.) Remembering his delicate, 'Ben, how did you cook this . . .?' as he picked shards of rock-hard rice out of his teeth still makes me smile. And it meant I was never asked to cook again, so result . . .?

My point is: the very act of walking removed our conversational filter. You're plodding along for miles with nothing else to do but chat. It removes the pressure of 'having a deep and meaningful' because you're *doing* something. You don't have to awkwardly avoid each other's eyes when you're busy trying not to fall down a crevasse, and you can always break any tension by screaming, 'LOOK AT THAT MASSIVE BADGER!' whenever you like.

Mental health is a tough thing to talk about for lots of reasons: you might not know what to say, you might not feel comfortable saying it, and you might not be in the right environment to say it. But the way most of us live nowadays actually leaves very little opportunity to broach those kinds of conversations. It's not like you'll be in the pub, watching football, and suddenly feel comfortable enough to drop in how you feel that your life isn't worth living and you have no hope for the future. Also, people have normalised their online lives to such an extent that it's considered acceptable to be on your phone constantly even while with your mates. It can feel as if they're not present, not engaged, and therefore not really interested. But you can't walk and scroll at the same time. Not for long anyway (which is why walking can be a great form of mindfulness, as, if you're fully focused on what's around you, you're entirely present in the moment).

As the messages from people at school continued to flood in (see previous chapter) – detailing loneliness, depression, anxiety, eating disorders, self-harm and all sorts – I realised that I was in a unique position: I was the only person who knew that all of these people were going through similar things. While that's no reason to crack open the fizz – 'Look! Everyone else is having a shocker too!' – knowing they weren't alone could make what they were going through feel less frightening. When two friends separately revealed to me that they were suffering from the same mental health issue, I remember thinking, *How powerful would it be if they could talk about it together?* I didn't want to betray their confidence, but I realised they were missing the opportunity and space to have that conversation and discover it for themselves. Couldn't I help to create that space, a kind of 'talking event'?

Let me be totally honest here: the idea of putting on an event wasn't simply to help everyone else, it was also to help me. I was still in desperate need of an escape. When I wasn't dealing with my grief, trauma, guilt and shame, I was revising for my bloody A-Levels. I'd never been one to worry too much about exams and I HATED revision. Urg. Even writing that word now fills me with memories of sheer, unadulterated boredom … and then stress. And then the stress of boredom. I would have rather assembled the whole school into the sports hall and delivered my rendition of 'Forever Friends' than revise. It's the fact that there's no natural end to it – that you can always do more. There isn't a point where you can shout, 'Job done!', slam your books shut, pat yourself on the back and wander off confident you know *everything* about maths. And, on top of hating studying anyway, I was really nervous now about being left alone with my thoughts – which is the definition of revision. The fact that I'm easily distracted would usually have meant my falling into endless YouTube rabbit holes (I'd start by watching a video tutorial on multiplying matrices and end up watching a video about the world's oceans spontaneously drying up), but this year was different and I knew those YouTube rabbit holes might get real dark real fast.

I also hoped that organising such a positive event would help to prove to myself that I was an okay person. As discussed in Chapter 3, the overwhelming guilt and shame I felt about everything meant that my sense of self-worth was pretty much non-existent. The belief that the very fabric of my being was intrinsically 'bad' had swallowed me up entirely. Maybe doing something 'good' could help to move the dial along and also help to pay back the debt I believed I owed Sam.

I didn't know it at the time, but there's a name for this: subli-mation. It's the idea that we take unwanted and unpleasant thoughts and turn them into positive action. As such, it's a well-known coping mechanism for grief and trauma. It's why you often hear about families that have lost loved ones starting charities or putting on events – it's a way of channelling all the sludge into something clearer, purer, better. (My parents did the same, setting up a charity in my brother's name in 2018: The Sam West Foundation.[1])

I was considering all this one February day while on the train to London. (Weirdly, I often have good ideas on public transport. Both there and in the shower. Imagine if I had a

SUBLIMATION IS THE IDEA THAT WE TAKE UNWANTED AND UNPLEASANT THOUGHTS AND TURN THEM INTO POSITIVE ACTION.

shower on a train – who knows what genius I'd come up with?) I sent a message to my best friends' Facebook group chat: *Does anyone want to do a walk to raise money for mental health charities?* Boom! The ball started rolling immediately, with everyone throwing ideas around. What should we call it? How far should we walk? Who would come? The excitement was contagious and within a couple of hours 'Project Walk to Talk' was born: a 10-day walk, starting at our school gates, heading through Canterbury and finishing in London: 200 kilometres, 10 days, two cities, one goal: make mental health a conversation.

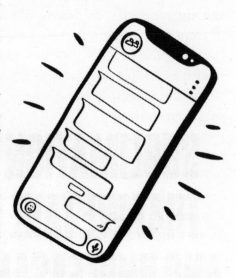

It was happening!

GOING DOWN LIKE A LEAD BALLOON

While researching the event, I made the horrendous mistake of google-image-searching 'mental illness'. Here's a recommendation: don't. It's not a laugh. All of the images were dark, sad and morbid, with dozens of variations of that standard pic of someone sitting alone in a corner with their head in their hands. Those kinds of pictures reinforce the belief that mental health as a subject is dark, lonely, depressing, frightening and silent and something to deal with on your own. That was the exact opposite vibe I wanted for Walk to Talk, so I immediately picked bright pink as the theme colour, bold and upbeat, and a camouflage print.

I thought pink camo symbolised what I wanted to achieve both on the walk and in general. The aim wasn't to remove the camouflage that people had constructed around their vulnerabilities, but rather to allow them to present it as something that exists. To say, 'Yes, here's my camouflage, here's my mask, and I'm not afraid to acknowledge them any more.' I didn't expect anyone to heal all their wounds on a walk – I knew putting on a pink camo t-shirt wasn't going to cure any illnesses – but I thought it might be the first time many people had even acknowledged their struggles or felt able to do so. There's a Japanese artform called kintsugi where broken pottery is repaired with precious metals, the cracks filled in with gold. It represents the idea that actually our faults are not weaknesses, or things to be ashamed of, but rather a part of our journey – things to be cherished and proud of. It's about embracing damage, and, in its own way, to me the pink camouflage represented those same values. Either way, it meant the t-shirts looked sick.

There was another intention behind choosing pink, as well as it being bright and bold. I thought it was also an interesting way of addressing the fragile foundation of toxic

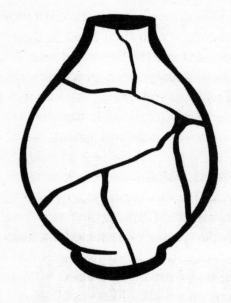

masculinity. Pink has long been associated with stereotypical concepts of femininity and has therefore been considered by many to be 'unmanly'. There are societal, historical and cultural contexts surrounding the colour, particularly in relation to the LGBTQ+ community, that I'm not best placed to go into, but I loved its associations with openness and inclusivity, and its challenges to stereotype and unconscious bias.

I really struggle to understand why we face such a barrier when it comes to male emotions and male mental health. Let's not dance around it: men have a real problem at the moment that we need to tackle. There is an expectation built upon traditional notions of masculinity that says men should act in a certain way. We have created a population that values stoicism and a fabricated illusion of toughness over the ability to cry, to be vulnerable and to not be okay. We value the unnatural suppression of emotion over the ability to be human. The suppression of emotions is celebrated as a sign of 'toughness', when actually recognising and expressing emotions is what's genuinely tough and takes courage. So let's once and for all

WE HAVE CREATED A POPULATION THAT VALUES STOICISM AND A FABRICATED ILLUSION OF TOUGHNESS OVER THE ABILITY TO CRY, TO BE VULNERABLE AND TO NOT BE OKAY.

put an end to this crap that 'we need tough men who can do strong men things' and instead change the conversation: 'strong men' are the ones who actually admit they're struggling. The old narrative is not only absolutely absurd but is claiming thousands of lives every year.

Even today, there are celebrities who will happily broadcast how important it is to be open about emotions and talk about mental health, while simultaneously advocating the idea that men need to be physically strong, hyper-productive and stoic. Here's news: there is NOTHING sexy or impressive about a man who has suppressed so many emotions during his life that it bubbles over into violence, aggression and the inability to have healthy relationships.

For most of my life I looked at emotions like they were the enemy, like they were something to stop. I buried feelings of sadness, loneliness or self-doubt. 'Tell me how you feel' people used to encourage, but to me that translated into the idea of being weak. A *real* man hides everything and just gets on with it. And then someone told me what 'expressing emotions' actually means: feeling what your brain is telling you to feel. Allowing your body to feel what it needs to at the time. Ta-da! That's it. That's the big secret. That really made me think differently about emotions: they're not your enemy, they're not trying to trip you up or make you into something you're not. They are simply necessary messages from your brain enabling you to process a specific event: *this* happened and you feel like *that* about it. If you feel sad, you're sad. If you're angry, you're angry. If you're happy, you're happy. At its root, it's really that

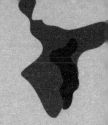

MALE SUICIDE: THE FACTS

While mental illness and suicide affect people of all genders, there is a particular need to highlight the sobering and scary reality that men are disproportionally dying from suicide in the UK:

* Seventy-five per cent of all suicides in the UK are men.[2]
* The largest cause of death for men under 50 is suicide.
* Men aged 40–49 have the highest suicide rates in the UK.
* Men are less likely to access psychological therapies than women: only 36 per cent of referrals to NHS talking therapies are for men.
* Higher rates of suicide are also found in minority communities, including gay men, war veterans, men from BAME backgrounds, and those with low incomes.[3]

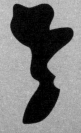
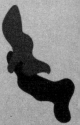

simple. Emotions are your body's way of processing what happens to you. You're meant to feel the feeling, acknowledge it, and let it run its course. Avoiding it or pretending it doesn't exist will only delay the inevitable crash and burn, adding anxiety about the avoidance on top. If you feel sad then yes, of course, it's okay to go out and do something to take your mind off it, but only as a temporary reprieve. If you're masking the emotion *all the time*, you must ask yourself why. The answer will probably be: *I don't think I can cope with the emotion when it comes. I can't deal with it.* The truth is: you absolutely *can* cope; you *can* deal with it. Yeah, it'll suck, but you'll feel better for having done it than you will waiting for it to get you – and then, because you've allowed it to happen, it'll pass.

The only way we can stop these feelings is by feeling them. You can try to delay them as much as you like, but eventually they have to be felt, which is why I use the word 'suppress'. Imagine every time you 'suppress' a feeling you blow it into a balloon. Each puff is an emotion you don't want to feel, such as:

- *rejection* when you don't get invited to an event;
- *vulnerability* when you consider telling a person that you have feelings for them;
- *disapproval* when you make a life choice that goes against expectations;
- *humiliation* when you don't get as many likes as your friend on Instagram.

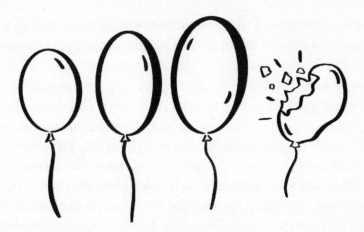

You can breathe every emotion you want to either ignore or avoid into the balloon. On the flip-side, whenever you do allow yourself to fully experience a mood, you let a bit of the air out. Now, as long as you're occasionally giving yourself time to check on that balloon and let some air out, you'll be okay . . . But, we all know what happens if you don't let any air out of the balloon at all. We all know what happens if you keep suppressing your emotions and huffing into that balloon pretending everything's just fine and dandy: the balloon gets bigger and bigger and BIGGER until eventually . . . BANG! All of that air – all of the shit you've stored up and suppressed and ignored – explodes over your head and you're *covered* in it. Not a pretty sight.

Think about your balloon for a moment (don't pretend you don't have one – we all do). How big is it right now? Have you been putting more air into it than letting air out? I'll be honest, right now, because I'm writing this book and processing a lot of shit, mine looks like a shrivelled little ball sack. Ha, not a phrase I ever thought I'd use, but we continue.

Being able to feel emotions when they arrive is a really important part of being human, but there can be a stigma associated with it. Talking can help to alleviate that stigma and also to help process whatever's going on, allowing your balloon to deflate. Unfortunately for men though, we just don't do this enough. Whether it's from how you're brought up, your peer group, popular culture, your social environment – whatever – it's true that, in general, men struggle more to open up.

Many guys don't want to let on that they have vulnerabilities or that they need anyone else: we are strong, independent men doing manly things! It's a false sense of personal superiority that makes talking about flaws or about things going wrong very hard. Like I said earlier, I don't remember where this personal sense of discomfort around emotional vulnerability and honesty came from, but there was definitely a sense of competition rather than community among other boys and men I knew growing up. Admitting that anything was wrong would be admitting you weren't coping and so were less of a man. Sam didn't want people to know how he was feeling and I didn't want people to know how I was feeling. I guess part of me wanted to appear like I was coping – in part through a hope that maybe it would actually trick me into thinking that I was – but also, when you have no idea how you're feeling, it's bloody intimidating trying to explain it to anyone else. How am I meant to articulate an emotion that is a mash-up of dozens and that I don't understand? Also, I'm a people-pleaser. I didn't want people to think I was lowering the mood or infecting everyone with negativity. I want to be liked and I want to like people, and being sad didn't mesh with that idea.

Don't get me wrong, I'm not saying that it's only men, or those who identify as men, who are struggling with mental health or mental health conversations. I'm saying that this is another aspect of the debate – one that has affected me personally and that we need to address. From my experience, there is a damaging narrative in which having mental health issues is considered a 'weakness', and it needs to be stamped out. I wanted Walk to Talk to address that, as well as everything else, especially as so many people reaching out to me were saying how I was the first young man they'd heard talking about this and that previously it had been a subject they'd considered off-limits to them.

Anyway, the pink camo t-shirts were designed in collaboration with a great company and would be part of a merch haul that we would sell before, during and after the walk to raise money for charity. We paid to get a couple of hundred printed and sat back thoroughly pleased with ourselves. Then, a couple of months later, I received a message from my mate who was in contact with the designer: 'Ben, we've got a problem . . .' and he showed me the text that we'd signed off: '200 kilometres. 10 days. 2 cities. 1 goal: Make mental health a conversion'.

'Yep. All good,' I said, waiting to hear the problem.

'Um, read the last word again,' he advised. 'Isn't that meant to say "conversation"?'

Oh fuck.

Maybe my primary school had been right about my linguistic ability after all. In my defence though, *dozens* of people saw that slogan and didn't say a word. We immediately phoned the printers and checked whether they'd started yet – and of course they had. There was only a couple of weeks to go by that point and they'd very nearly finished our entire order.

Our next idea was to figure out how we could make mental health a conversion. There must be a way! Could we make it rugby themed? No, ridiculous. The whole lot had to be reprinted. Luckily for us though, the new (correct) batch arrived in time and people couldn't get enough of them. (I actually sometimes still see people out running wearing one of the tees or at the gym repping Walk to Talk merch, which is really nice.)

INSTAGRAM ACCOUNTS THAT PROMOTE POSITIVE MENTAL HEALTH CONVERSATIONS (NOT CONVERSIONS)

One of the keys to good mental health is sculpting your environment into a safe and supportive space – and one of the environments many of us spend *a lot* of time in is the world of social media. Think of your social media accounts like your home. Who are you happy to let in? Who do you grudgingly grant access? And who are you shouting at through the letterbox to go away? I talk more about how to create a positive social media space for yourself on page 206, but below are some accounts that I think you should let into your social home because they're always welcome in mine.

@iambenwest (obvs)
@chessiekingg
@mattzhaig
@mattjohnsons
@IAMWHOLE
@giveusashoutinsta
@hopevirgo_
@mrjonnybenjamin
@thebookofman
@wearebey0nd

@humenorg
@lukeambleruk
@poornabell
@jonolanc
@scarrednotscared
@dralexgeorge
@drjulie
@joetracini
@catherine_benfield

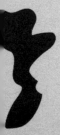

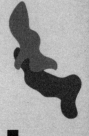

RUNNING OFF MY A-LEVELS

For the next five months I *threw* myself into organising this walk. I couldn't get enough of it. I thought about why people weren't talking, making a list of all the barriers I could think of and then trying to come up with a way of tackling each and every one during the event. The whole thing would be a waste of time if everyone spent 10 days chatting about the weather or their favourite protein shake. We asked several organisations and charities for leaflets that we could hand out, providing different mental health advice and support. One was to parents on how to start talking to their children about the subject; another was directed at the people suffering; and another was for friends and partners. Handing those out at the start would establish our intention head-on: we were there to talk about mental health. It would be expected and encouraged.

My friends and I mapped out a 200 kilometre route – from Cranbrook, Kent, to Parliament Square, London – that would take 10 days to complete, starting on 27 August 2018. Anyone who had signed up for a 'ticket' (the event was free, of course, but we needed to keep track of numbers), would cover approximately 20 kilometres a day, then either head home and travel to the next start point the next morning, or stay somewhere en route.

By the beginning of August, everything was ready to go and me and my friend Johnny (who I've known since I was three and who had been part of the Walk to Talk team since the beginning), had a meeting with our local MP to try to drum up some extra support. We were shocked when she started singing our praises, saying she wanted to book a room in the Houses of Parliament for us all to celebrate at the end. Back in the car, Johnny and I screamed like we'd won the Lottery. We'd put in so much hard work that being promised a proper finale felt like a testament to the idea and a positive omen.

A week or so before, I decided to run the route, just to check that it was all legit and I wasn't about to lead hundreds of people into a swamp or off a cliff. I'm not a professional runner or anything (imagine if I actually was and just slid that in here like, 'Surprise! I just ran five marathons back to back!') but I found running very therapeutic and earlier that year I'd surprised myself by going out for a jog and going just a little bit further ... and a little bit further still ... until I ended up running a half-marathon. The thought of trying to run this route appealed to me; let's see what I could do. I didn't put too much pressure on myself, just running or walking as far as I could each day, and I ended up completing the first four days of the walk's route. I found it really peaceful and it reassured me that our plan was fine. I mean, apart from the random river I found on Day 3, smack-bang in the middle of the path. (I can't actually remember now if I changed that bit or if everyone ended up having to wade through it. I wasn't there that day, for reasons you'll soon discover.)

So, everything was ready – all that was left was the walk itself. Time to sit back, relax, safe in the knowledge that surely nothing could possibly go wrong now. Right?

PEG-LEGS AND TINY PUPILS

People really connected with the idea of the walk – far more than we'd anticipated. Despite the fact that lots had signed up, in my mind I figured maybe 10 or 20 would actually show up on the day. So, imagine my shock to find 150 people waiting at the start on 27 August.

The buzz was incredible and I couldn't help feeling super-proud – all of this was the result of a single random idea I'd had on a train in February! A couple of us said a few words at the start, reiterating the point of the day – to talk to those around you openly and honestly about mental health – then we handed out the leaflets and got cracking. A pink army walking through tiny Kent villages and down little lanes; all in our tees, with pink wristbands and face paint – it was an epic sight. My dog, Tippy, even had her own t-shirt.

The only hiccup on that first day was when we arrived at one field and, Kent being Kent, it was full of cows. Now, I'm not sure whether it was the pink or whether they were just feeling particularly happy that day, but these were the friendliest cows you've ever seen. No one could get through the gate as the cows all crowded round it trying to introduce themselves. How do you get 150 people through a field of cows without anyone getting trampled? I have no idea, is the honest answer, but, we did – albeit a remarkably long time later.

We were so happy at the end of Day 1. It was great fun, people enjoyed it, we didn't get majorly lost and no one got trampled by cows. Someone did break their finger on a hay bale at kilometre 10 (nope, I've no idea how either), but that was it. Result! To celebrate, lots of us headed to the local pub, which had a live band. I'm a *dreadful* dancer (which is annoying because one of my closest mates is officially one of the best ballroom dancers in the world. I've lost count of the number of times Max has tried to teach me to dance, saying, 'Ben, it's easy – just do this', and I'll watch blankly as he does things with his feet that I didn't know feet could do). But we were on a high and dancing was the order of the day, so I 'danced'. A sudden shooting pain in my foot taught me the error of my ways though, and I retreated back to the safety of my seat ... where my foot started to swell up. I could walk, but certainly not well. I'm not sure where I stand with the law here, to be honest, so I'm sorry, officer, but I drove everyone back in my manual car that evening using only my left foot. Anyone familiar with manual cars will realise that's not ideal and is definitely much harder than it sounds.

The thought that I might have seriously injured myself was too ridiculous to contemplate so I went to bed, convinced that I'd wake up in the morning and it would all be fine. Not so!

When I woke up, my foot was huge. Monstrous. I couldn't walk on it at all. Not ideal when you have *no* choice but to walk another 170 kilometres over the next nine days. Not completing the charity walk I had created because I'd somehow broken my foot while doing the Charleston in a random pub in the middle of a field was not an option. So I dusted off the crutches I'd kept from when I broke my ankle (yep, from when I was 10 years old – we'd tried to give them back to the hospital but they wouldn't take them) and decided to continue that way. A few kilometres taught me the stupidity of that brainwave. Crutches weren't designed for long distances, especially off-road – my palms were purple, my arms and shoulders were on fire, and I was so exhausted I couldn't have talked if someone paid me to. Walk to Talk, my arse. It had become more like Hop and Groan. I had no choice but to stop and let everyone carry on without me, and that was awful. I'd spent so long planning, and it meant so much to me, that watching it unfold without my taking part was tragic. Luckily, my team was fantastic and everyone knew what they were doing, so it didn't make a huge difference to the walk that I wasn't there; it just made a huge difference to me.

To keep my spirits up, I made it a priority to sort myself out so I could re-join again as soon as possible. The first stop? My favourite place: A&E. (I should have an A&E loyalty card: collect five x-rays and get an MRI scan for free.) The good news was: my foot wasn't broken or fractured, but no one knew what was actually wrong with it; the doctor's best guess was that I'd torn a ligament from repetitive strain (nice). I rang up a physio friend, Liz, and screamed, 'LIZ. I HAVE TO WALK AND I HAVE TO WALK NOW. WHAT CAN YOU DO?', and she immediately understood the assignment. Knowing that physiotherapy wouldn't provide an instant solution, she suggested something called an iWalk. This is a genius contraption that's basically an 'armless crutch' that sits on the bottom of your leg like a peg-leg! We very nearly went for that pirate look, but it wouldn't arrrr-rive in time (sorry), so the quickest and easiest option was to ask my GP for the strongest painkillers available.

By this point, I'd missed out on Day 3, but would make it for Day 4. Arriving at the start on crutches, I necked a couple of the magic painkillers and – honestly, I'm just going to tell it like it was – threw my crutches down and started run-hopping around the car park with a coat over my head shouting, 'Peekaboo!' at random strangers. People were arriving at my event, to walk my route and raise money for my cause, and I was *off my face* on codeine. Oh, boy. My friends kept telling me, 'Ben, your pupils are *tiny*', and I'd grin inanely at them, walking on clouds.

But those painkillers worked because miles turned into marathons and days turned into, well, 10 days, and eventually around 50 of us staggered into London's Parliament Square, totally elated. We'd finished! It was an incredible feeling, our pink army running across rush-hour roads, cheering and celebrating because we had made it.

Our MP came good and we ended the walk with a reception in the Houses of Parliament. There were speeches, a lot to drink, and even a surprise letter from Theresa May, the prime minister at the time. But what meant more to me than any of that, what I was most proud of, was that not only had we raised £15,000, but that over the 10 days, 450 people had taken part, and we'd achieved our aim of getting people to talk. People told me how they'd spoken to their loved ones about their situations for the first time; parents revealed they'd discussed their concerns with their children; and I even had people tell me that they'd started counselling afterwards. Hell, I even received a card that I still keep by my bed thanking the team for saving someone's life.

We started Walk to Talk with the aim of encouraging more open conversations about mental health and I have absolutely no doubt that it worked. Both for those who were there and for those who were affected afterwards. During the walk itself, I found it remarkable how pretty much immediately people started talking really candidly about mental health. Someone came because their son had anorexia (he wasn't on the walk himself) and they were there to support the cause – they didn't actually think it would change or affect their personal situation in any big way. Yet, soon afterwards, they felt able to speak to their son as a family about his condition for the first time. The walk had normalised the subject for them, made it less awkward and less taboo.

I was proud beyond words – and that pride came at a time when I had very little. Pulling off Walk to Talk finally allowed me to admit that maybe I'd done okay by Sam after all. As much as that walk helped others, it helped me most of all.

Coming down from that buzz led to the inevitable question: 'What next?' The more involved I'd got with the event and the more conversations I'd had with people, the more I started realising the scale of what we were dealing with and how much needed to change. I felt a real responsibility to continue campaigning and to try my hardest to affect change – not just locally but nationally. When I'd been doing CPR on Sam, I'd told him that I wasn't going to stop; that I was going to do everything it took to help him. That was the promise I made and, after the walk, I knew that promise extended far beyond that one moment. I saw what was going on for people in Sam's position. I knew how much they were hurting, but how little energy they had to campaign for change themselves. But I had the energy. I could do it for them.

If not me, then who? If not now, then when?

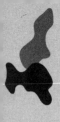
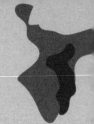

TIPS ON STARTING YOUR OWN MENTAL HEALTH CONVERSATION

Talking about mental health is *hard.* No one enjoys having difficult conversations; they're sad and, well, difficult. We therefore tend to ignore warning signs within ourselves and in others because we don't want to open a Pandora's box. Talking about feelings makes us vulnerable, like an onion that's had its outer layer removed, and that's scary.

However, it's one thing to decide you do actually want to talk – it's quite another to have the opportunity to do so. There are obviously systemic societal issues we can get into (and oh, we will), but the advice here is for people looking to create opportunities to talk in a smaller, more immediate and intimate way.

IF YOU'RE WORRIED ABOUT SOMEONE YOU KNOW

Assume you are the only person who is worried and reach out. It can be easy to think, 'They're probably talking to someone else' or 'their partner/pal/colleague/boss probably has it handled.' They might not, so do it. Imagine you later discovered you were the only one who did . . . and you almost didn't.

Within your message, emphasise how *you* want to talk. Too often we put the onus on the person who's hurting to reach out, which is incredibly difficult for them. People suffering from mental illness

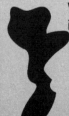

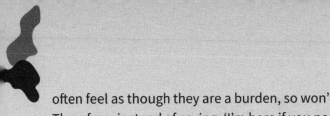

often feel as though they are a burden, so won't make the move. Therefore, instead of saying, 'I'm here if you need me, let me know', say, 'If you think it would be helpful, I'd love to chat.' It's a simple and subtle difference that considerably changes the tone of your message. You're saying you *want* to chat rather than that you're simply available to.

Sending a message is fine. You don't have to call them, rock up at their house or make a grand gesture. Often people don't feel able to talk at a particular moment, so a message allows them to read, digest and respond in their own time.

Follow up a while later and reiterate your offer. It's not being pushy; it'll show you really mean it. This time, invite them around for a brew or ask if they want to go for a walk. Having something to do while you're talking is a good way of making things more comfortable. I have a phrase I use: 'cup of tea, 1, 2, 3'. Tea and coffee are GIFTS in this situation. When we're nervous or uncomfortable, holding a warm mug and sipping on a warm drink is comforting. Once the mug is in hand, count to three in your head (not out loud, that would be weird) and say something like the following . . .

'Is there anything you'd like to get off your chest?' or 'What's going on?' Choosing such phrases instead of 'How are you?' immediately addresses the elephant in the room. 'How are you?' or 'Alright?' are often used as variations of 'Hello' and, culturally, people aren't always expected to answer truthfully (many of us would be very surprised if they did). Because of this, it can be hard to tell if they're genuine questions or not. Asking instead, 'Is there anything you'd like to get off your chest?' makes it clear you do really want a proper answer.

》

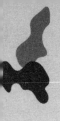

You don't have to 'fix' what's wrong. Most people want to help and offer solutions when they know someone's struggling – I certainly do. I'm the sort of person who will hijack a conversation and dish out all the advice. Sure, that's okay at times, but, first, it's not your job to 'fix' anything, second, it might put you off speaking to them if you're not sure how to 'help', and third, it might put them off speaking to you if they think you're just going to barrage them with suggestions.

No one expects you to solve anything. If you found someone who'd just had a stroke, you'd ask if they're okay even though you're not a physician, right? Well, same goes here: no one's going to leap out demanding your psychotherapy qualifications for just *listening*. The single best thing you can do to help is listen. Ask open-ended questions like, 'How does that make you feel?' and let them say whatever they need to say.

Don't be scared to be vulnerable yourself. A good way to make someone feel comfortable talking about their own emotions is to talk about yours. Set the tone and make them feel safe, by telling them about what's going on with you, which gives them permission to open up too. It was only when I started talking about my situation that I started receiving messages from other people. That wasn't a coincidence: vulnerability is infectious. You obviously don't have to spill everything or hijack the chat, but simply setting a precedent by admitting that you have struggled is powerful.

I will also note here that living with or loving someone who is suffering from a mental illness can be exhausting, draining and incredibly demanding, so if you need support yourself then make sure you reach out too. Remember, the very best counsellors all have counsellors of their own.

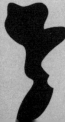

IF YOU'RE STRUGGLING YOURSELF AND WANT TO REACH OUT

Given I've admitted actively avoiding conversations about my own mental health, this might sound a bit 'do as I say, not as I do', but there are things that have made it much easier for me to open up, and that have been relayed to me by others:

* Practice makes perfect. Knowing you're going to have to reveal something big can be terrifying. 'How do I start the conversation? What are they going to say? What if I stumble and fall down a pothole?' Build up your confidence by practising. Yes, that sounds weird, but trust me. Do a role play and act out the conversation, literally saying it all out loud, picturing the scene. Where are you? How are you standing (i.e. shoulders back, chin up)? What are you wearing (something that makes you feel brave)? What are you going to say? What are they going to say? Visualising it like this, actually *seeing* the conversation happen in your head, will make it much less daunting.

* Take control of 'cup of tea, 1, 2, 3'. Invite someone you love over for a brew, hug your mug, count to three, and just say it. Alternatively, invite the person for a walk.

* Reach out to an objective professional or an anonymous helpline. Someone you don't know who you may feel more comfortable opening up to. Please see the resources on page 281.

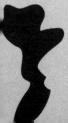
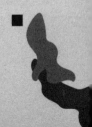

TAKEAWAYS

- Create your own mini Walk to Talk by asking someone to join you on a stroll, whether you're the one looking to unload or suspect they might be. Walking limits the pressure and intensity of a face-to-face chat and removes conversational filters.

- Remember: giving people the opportunity to talk about mental health is far more useful than simply telling them how important it is to talk. Create safe spaces however you can – and tell someone that you *want* to help rather than that you are available to do so.

- If you are nervous about starting a conversation about your own mental health, you can practise it first to build confidence. Visualisation is a powerful tool. Try it!

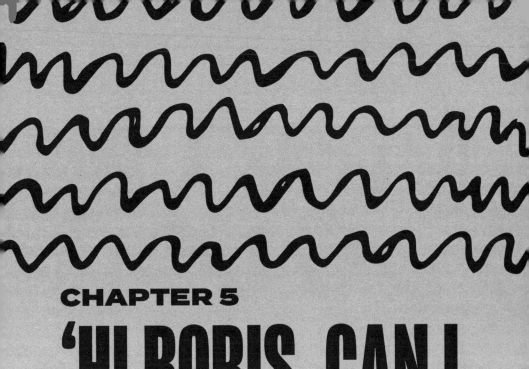

CHAPTER 5

'HI BORIS, CAN I HAVE A WORD?'

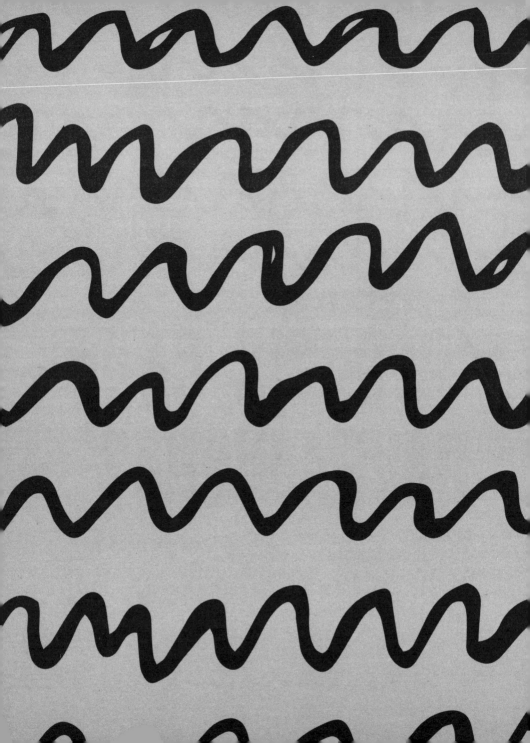

'Why should teachers be given the responsibility of looking after their students' mental health?' the online comment read. I stared at it, dumbfounded. It was part of an ongoing social media discussion I'd started about the importance of teachers being trained in mental health as standard. 'The burden of that added responsibility is nothing compared to the burden of having to see the empty seat in your classroom left by the student you never had the tools to help.' This answer, from a teacher invested in the topic, was swift and powerful and brought a lump to my throat.

It was September 2018, just after Walk to Talk, and I was deep-diving into a subject that had come up multiple times in conversations with school staff: the lack of training they received in mental health and mental health support. After Sam's death, I'd been shocked by the number of teachers at our school who told me that they lacked the expertise to know how or when to step in. They wanted to help, they cared (no one signs up to be a teacher if they hate kids . . . I hope), but they hadn't been trained to spot the signs or know how to activate a support process.

I thought that was batshit.

When you're young, you assume that adults generally, and particularly those in positions of power, have things sorted. You figure that society has rumbled on long enough that at least some of the people leading it must know what they're doing. It can therefore come as a real shock – especially at 18 years old – to discover that many of them don't. And, not only that, but that long-standing systemic failures exist that everyone is aware of, but that no one's doing anything to fix.

My response to discovering that teachers didn't know how to navigate their students' emotional needs was a big fat WTAF? I'd believed that Sam was getting the necessary help; that the adults in charge of such things – the teachers, counsellors, doctors, NHS, and so on – would be sorting shit out. To that end, I guess I also believed that his death was an anomaly, that he died *despite* being offered all possible support and understanding. To realise that this wasn't the case was one of those punch-you-in-the-gut moments. Like, wait, what – this is unacceptable, right? Then why aren't we all fuming about it?

Don't get me wrong – I'm not blaming Sam's teachers. I'm sure they did the best they could. I'm blaming the fact that, at the time, *it wasn't compulsory for teachers to know anything about mental health at all.*

In 2017, the government announced a green paper[1] (a tentative report and consultation document that may or may not be taken into law) that claimed they 'will ensure that a member of staff in every primary and secondary school receives mental health awareness training'. My thoughts on this were, first: *'a* member of staff?' Really? One person per school wasn't close to being okay. You're telling me that one person in a whole school can take responsibility for spotting the warning signs of struggle in hundreds of students and/or be responsible for training their colleagues to do so? Allow me a big laugh. Thank you. Moving on to the second problem: that simply wasn't a sustainable model. Cherry-picking certain teachers (how? who?), taking them out of work to attend a course, only to return to school and be responsible for the mental health of the entire institution? Why not put the onus on teacher-training organisations to integrate the training so that every newly qualified teacher comes to school with those skills already, therefore slowly filling up the profession with people who are trained in mental health first aid? Now *that* is sustainable.

I couldn't believe this shit. More so when teachers explained to me how student mental health was a heavily stigmatised topic within leadership and that schooling in general was (and still is) so deep-rooted in tradition and so riddled with bureaucracy that accepting responsibility for more than just academic education came with a lot of resistance.

So, not only were teachers untrained in it, but kids weren't getting taught about it. There were *no* mandatory lessons assigned to the topic in either primary or secondary education. At this point (in 2018), mental wellbeing wasn't even an essential part of PSHE (personal, social, health and economic) lessons. (It would become mandatory in September 2020, but, due to Covid, schools were given a grace period to enact changes to the curriculum until September 2021, when they had to start teaching it.) And, to be totally honest, PSHE classes were treated as a bit of a joke by my class anyway. Take sex education for example: those classes were *always* taught by someone flustered and awkward as hell, who'd stutter and stumble over descriptions of sex acts while we threw massive bright-blue dildos around the classroom and put condoms over our heads, blowing them up with our noses. That kind of atmosphere didn't bode well for discussions about mental health, and if teachers weren't trained in it or comfortable with it, the lessons ran the risk of further stigmatising mental illness, putting us into a worse situation than we were already. (This supposition of mine was confirmed when, in 2019, the PSHE Association itself stated that: 'robust PSHE education is rarely included in initial teacher-training education (ITE), meaning many teachers will have had very little, if any, training on delivering this potentially sensitive subject area'. It even went on to say that, 'taught badly, PSHE can do more harm than good'.[2])

It is a default defence response to push away, laugh at or downplay things we don't understand or find frightening – imagine what a rowdy class of kids laughing about anxiety could do to the person in the corner who's got GAD.

WHAT ARE SCHOOLS FOR, IF NOT THIS?

In my opinion, a school's main purpose must be to prepare young people for adulthood. How did the focus become so much about data and exam results? Schools are exam factories, students passing down a production line before being churned out into higher education or work. How does that measure the quality, strength and resilience of a person? In the grand scheme of things, academic ability is not a sensible assessment of what it means to be a functioning, valuable and valued adult.

It's fair to say that I was exceptionally pissed off about the nature of modern education. I thought the state of it was so dire that it was claiming people's lives, costing the economy billions of pounds (in misspent funding and the loss of future earnings through mental illness), and causing totally preventable suffering to millions. The fact that students weren't being taught about stress, anxiety, sadness, depression, worries, unconscious bias, confirmation bias, prejudice, self-worth, confidence and body image as a major part of the curriculum was a colossal mistake.

People often asked me, 'What is mental health?', and my answer was simple: it's what makes you *you*. Everything you've ever thought, everything you've ever done, your personality, memories, values and your dreams for the future – all of it is dependent on, and influenced by, how you feel about both yourself and your environment. Mental health dictates the decisions you make and how you interact with the world. Now, tell me if I'm wrong here, but surely that's an important thing to cover straight off the bat at school? And to anyone who says, 'But primary school students are too young for that', I would kindly like to direct them to these stats:

- Of children aged nine to 12, 1,225 were admitted to hospital for intentional self-harm or intentional self-poisoning[3] (which are classed separately) in 2019.
- Studies have shown that certain mental health conditions, in particular anxiety disorders, can have an onset age of as young as four years old.[4]
- Half of all mental ill-health starts by age 15, and 75 per cent develops by age 18.[5] This means that a huge number of kids learn about mental health as a patient from a doctor, rather than as a student from a teacher. How fucked is that?

THIS MEANS THAT A HUGE NUMBER OF KIDS LEARN ABOUT MENTAL HEALTH AS A PATIENT FROM A DOCTOR, RATHER THAN AS A STUDENT FROM A TEACHER.

During my own time at school I heard the words 'mental health' on a few occasions, usually in some abstract way that didn't register. We had a couple of guest assemblies and presentations on it, but then we also had guest assemblies on the techniques of French pantomime, so, you know, who cares? Kids value and prioritise what they are taught to value and prioritise. If they only learn about mental health from some random woman dressed like your nan who's given the same amount of airtime as a guy the next week discussing foreign theatre, that says a lot about where it's going to rank on a kid's give-a-shit-o-meter. My utter confusion and misunderstanding of Sam's diagnosis is testament to my ignorance – and I was 17. How did I get to 17 knowing *nothing* about what was happening to him and to so many others?

We needed – and still need – a system that prioritises prevention over reaction and education over medication. We had to recognise the role that schools play in teaching us not only how to read, write, add and subtract, but also how to feel, how to interpret thoughts in a safe and healthy way, and how to process difficult and uncomfortable emotions. I knew that if we were going to get serious about mental health education we needed to teach it from a young age, and it should be taught by people the students trusted (i.e. their teachers, not some stranger) who was confident in the subject.

Within mental health conversations, we talk a lot about the support that either is or isn't available, disregarding two important points:

To get to the stage where support is offered or a diagnosis made, someone's had to either recognise and accept something is wrong and seek help themselves (which obviously doesn't always happen). Or, an external figure has had to recognise it and intervene (which again, doesn't always happen).

A lot of mental illness diagnoses could be avoided entirely if we prioritised prevention and education.

Yes, some mental health problems are genetic, hereditary or situational, meaning prevention isn't an option – but being educated on coping mechanisms certainly is. If a young person was taught how to recognise patterns in their own emotional responses and their behaviour, learn how feelings and behaviour are intrinsically linked, as well as coping strategies for when things get rough, it could literally save lives.

Realising this in September 2018, my new project was a no-brainer: start a petition for teachers to be trained in mental health – both in spotting the signs of a student struggling and in knowing how to ensure they get the support they need. I went onto www.change.org and set up a petition called: 'Save Our Students: Make Mental Health First Aid a Compulsory Part of Teacher Training'.

'Mental health first aid' is exactly what it says on the tin. Similar to physical first aid, it gives you a basic understanding of what to do should a situation arise where you're concerned about someone's welfare. Teachers trained in this would learn what causes mental illnesses, be able to recognise signs of someone struggling, and know the best ways of offering help and signposting support. What mental health first aid *won't* do is give someone the qualifications to, or the expectation that they can, provide clinical care, in the same way that taking a first aid course doesn't enable you to conduct open heart surgery. What it *does* do is equip someone to get the necessary help more quickly to a person who is suffering and to provide them with support to try and stop their condition getting worse before they get professional help.

THE RUNAWAY PETITION AND ALL THAT FOLLOWED

My aim in creating the petition wasn't only to induce change and implement mandatory training; it was, in large part, simply to raise awareness of the fact that teachers weren't prepared to deal with mental illness and mental health issues. That, if confronted by a sobbing student, a teacher might not have the faintest idea what to do other than pat them on the head, recommend they drink more water, or give them one of those damp blue tissues that are used on everything from grazes to fractured limbs. I guessed that, like me, many people simply assumed that they were trained. After all, mental health was such a big deal – the biggest threat to the life of a teenager[6] – so how could they not be?

To confirm again: I wasn't having a go at teachers at all. I was having a go at the systemic failures that allowed things to get to this stage. Many teachers were totally supportive of the petition and the intention behind it, and, in fact, many schools are absolutely smashing it when it comes to mental health training and support. They haven't waited for laws to enforce training, but have taken the initiative themselves, opting to train staff in mental health first aid and provide on-site counsellors and specialists, either independently or in partnership with external organisations. To those schools: big up.

But for the others, at the mercy of an outdated system – well. One teacher told me how bizarre he found it that he had to know how to administer an EpiPen, in case a student went into anaphylactic shock, but nothing about what to do if a student was self-harming. How many students suffer anaphylactic shock every year, you may ask? Well, according to NHS Digital Figures for 2018 to 2019:[7]

- There were 728 hospital admissions in England for children between the ages of 11 and 18 suffering anaphylactic shock.
- During the same time period, 18,895 young people between the ages of 13 and 17 were admitted to hospital for intentional self-harm or intentional self-poisoning in England alone.[8]
- On top of that, in the same period, 196 people aged between 10 and 19 died from suicide,[9] making it the leading cause of death for adolescents in England and Wales.[10]

Obviously, I wasn't saying we should stop teachers being trained in how to respond to allergic reactions. I was saying clearly we should *also* train them in how to respond to mental health issues. The numbers don't lie. It *had* to change and it pissed me off that politicians kept proudly broadcasting how important they thought mental health was, and 'raising awareness', and then just brazenly ignored it within the most important institution to do with kids' growth, health and safety.

The petition reached a hundred signatures within hours. And then a thousand. A couple of weeks later: five thousand. At that point a woman called Rima from change.org reached out to me, explaining how the platform supported what we were calling for and wanted to suggest a few things we could do to maximise the petition's reach. I hung up on that call feeling immensely excited – this was happening: we could potentially influence actual systemic change. I kept thinking about Sam, and all the other people who'd contacted me saying they felt suicidal, and wondering how many would never have got to that place if someone had intervened early. If support had been offered sooner or at all. To me, this was more than just an online petition; it felt like it was the difference between life and death: the change that people's lives depended on – and they didn't even realise.

A few days after that call with Rima, I woke up to a text message from a friend: 'BEN, go look at the petition RIGHT NOW!' I blearily logged on, blinked, rubbed my eyes like some hammy cartoon character, and looked again: twenty thousand signatures. I blinked and refreshed the page. Twenty-two thousand signatures. I refreshed again: twenty-five thousand signatures. The petition was exploding and messages of support were flooding in! Soon we had sixty thousand signatures. SIXTY THOUSAND! I couldn't believe it – we had the backing of sixty thousand people who believed in this change.

To be totally honest, I hadn't actually thought it would work. Don't get me wrong – I always thought it was a good idea – I one hundred per cent believed it was something that should happen, but I'd had very little hope that the petition would receive a significant number of signatures. I knew hundreds of petitions were sent into cyberspace and were quickly lost to the ether. I'd figured that as long as I got the word out and made more people aware of the situation, that was good enough. But that all changed after seeing the names roll in day after day. We were clearly onto something – we had struck a nerve – and I was determined to do everything possible to keep that momentum going.

INSTAGRAM INFLUENCE(R)

It was around this time that my journey on social media really started. Instagram became a tool by which I could raise awareness of, and direct people to, the petition. I put a huge amount of time and effort into growing my presence on that platform. I mean a *huge* amount of time and effort. I made it my goal to gain a hundred new followers every day, so a thousand new followers every 10 days, meaning I'd amass that magic ten thousand figure within six weeks. (Ten thousand is the 'magic figure' because your follower count becomes assessed by the letter 'k' rather than zeroes, so 10k, and you're given the ability to add web links to your stories. This sounds totally banal, but in terms of reach, it's important.) I worked on this growth each day: posting, interacting, conducting takeovers – you name it, I did it. Why? Because I recognised that, for better or worse, social media was where most of my peers were connecting and so that was where my message was best placed. And, the more I grew my audience and the more I put myself out there, the more I realised that I actually had something to say. People were listening to me – not only listening, but really supporting what I was doing. It reaffirmed what I was trying to do and reassured me that the change I was pushing for was entirely necessary and long overdue.

At this point, I was still coming to terms with what had happened in my life. The pain, the trauma and the grief were all still there, still thrumming along under the surface. Social media for me became a place where I could channel that and be vulnerable without judgement. There was a community of people who either felt the way I did, felt the way Sam had, or who knew someone who did and cared. This vulnerability around my own mental health opened the door once again for people to talk to me about their own experiences. With every conversation, my concern for the future and my desperation for change grew. It felt as though I'd been woken up out of this cushy dream to find the world on fire and no one was doing anything about it. 'ARE YOU SEEING THIS SHIT?' I wanted to shout. And so I did. And the resounding answer coming back to me was: Yes, we're seeing it too.

Finding that outlet also exposed me to the sheer scale of the mental health crisis affecting the country. The more people I reached, the more stories I heard that backed up the rapidly evolving picture I was formulating of the shitshow we were all in. I realised this was impacting *millions* of people (not all of whom were in my inbox, thank God – although at times it sure felt like they were). What also became abundantly clear was how *exhausting* mental illness can be to those who suffer from it. People told me how hard they found it simply to get out of bed in the morning, let alone campaign for changes around mental health education and training. I saw I was in a unique position: I not only had the energy to take on this challenge, but I was coming at it from an alternative perspective – that of someone who's never had a mental illness. I'm not experiencing this personally yet can still understand the urgency and importance of it, so why can't politicians and decision makers? It's easy for people to dismiss those personally invested in a particular issue: 'Of course you care about this; you're in it. The rest of us aren't. Goodbye now.' But it's harder to also dismiss those who can see what a mess it is from the outside – you can't dismiss *everyone*. I felt like I owed it to those in Sam's position to do my very best to say what they wanted said, and to fight for the change they needed.

It goes back to the point I made at the very beginning of this book: I'm lucky that I haven't had to experience what mental illness feels like. It's that luck which makes me want to do what I do – because being lucky doesn't give me, or anyone else, permission not to care.

AEROSPACE ENGINEERING? SOUNDS GREAT. SIGN ME UP.

On 15 September 2018, I started university. So here's the thing: I am shit at maths. I just about scraped through my A-Level exam in the subject with A LOT of help. I'm not just saying that – in my mock paper, I got a U – so you can likely spot the problem when I tell you that the course I'd opted for was Aerospace Engineering. Yes, literal rocket science. What on earth was I thinking?!

My first lecture was two hours of hardcore, incomprehensible maths. The kind of maths you'll see in a meme because it's so insanely complicated. I left that lecture laughing my arse off because I'd barely understood a word of it. It was clear from the outset that my course was not going to be what I'd imagined. Yes, I'd always had an interest in planes and flight, but I think it says it all that, after a couple of years of studying the subject, I'm still not exactly sure how planes fly. Magic, right? Let's just say it's a good thing this book isn't titled, *The Principles of Modern Aviation*, because it would be exceptionally short. (If you're struggling with your own course, by the way, please see the tips on page 212.)

TIPS FOR MANAGING SOCIAL ANXIETY

We've all felt it. Whether it's a dreaded public speaking event or casual drinks in the pub, social anxiety is something that happens to even the most extroverted people. And yes, it happens to me. In my experience, we project what we believe other people are thinking onto ourselves: e.g. 'Urg, I look awful. I bet other people are thinking it too. I bet they're thinking my jumper is a terrible colour. God, why did I choose to wear this? I should go home.' Anxiety around socialising is often caused by what you're telling yourself other people are thinking, when in reality, (a) YOU'RE NOT A MIND-READER, and (b) they're not thinking that at all (they're probably worrying about what *you're* thinking about *them*).

Here are my top tips for dealing with it:

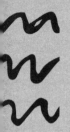

* Notice that you're feeling anxious, *say it* and then *thank the anxiety for being there*. No, I'm not on codeine; I mean it. You need to name it to tame it: 'Okay, I'm feeling anxious. My fingertips are tingling and I've got butterflies. Thanks for looking out for me, anxiety, but I'm safe and I'm not going to get hurt.' This will calm your body down (see page 219) and make you feel more in control. It's easy to bully yourself – 'Snap out of it!' – when all that does is make you feel worse. The anxiety is only trying to help you; trying to keep you safe by making you run away. However, that's actually the least helpful thing you can do, because if you keep avoiding the

thing you're scared of, you're not giving yourself the chance to disprove your fear.

* Offer to hand out the snacks or drinks at an event where that's not weird (i.e. in someone's home). It gives you a natural way of introducing yourself and also an excuse to leave a conversation: 'Hi, I'm Ben, Sarah's friend. Would you like some crisps? How do you know Sarah?' Right, I've got to go and deliver some more of these. Catch you later!'

* Pick a group of four or five people to join and listen to for a while. Much less pressure than one-on-one.

* Discuss something that's relevant to the event so everyone can join in: 'Look at that thing over there. What do you think?/Have you been here before?/I just got shat on by a seagull. Has that ever happened to you? Isn't it meant to be good luck?'

* Choose events where you know you won't feel overwhelmed – i.e. a cinema trip, a pub quiz or walking tour – where the onus isn't on you making small talk but on discussing the activity.

* It is easier said than done, and practice makes perfect, but changing your internal dialogue from super self-critical to calm and in control is a really good step towards being able to tackle those anxious moments. If your anxiety is affecting your day-to-day life though, and stopping you from doing things you'd usually do, it could be a sign that you have an anxiety disorder. Please talk to your doctor for more advice.

»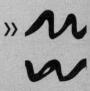

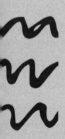

* If you see someone else who may be suffering from social anxiety, great, you're in a position to help make things easier for them:
  - Invite them to join a bigger group of people who are already chatting (not making them the focus, so they can just listen in at first).
  - Take the lead with the conversation.
  - Don't be scared to try to be funny; laughter defuses tension.
  - Ask if they want to help you make some drinks or pass the snacks. Having a role can take the pressure off.
  - Don't draw attention to their insecurity – i.e. 'What are you doing standing over there alone? Don't be shy! Oh, your face just went really red.'
  - Don't talk for them. As much as you think you might be helping out, you may make them feel more isolated and are removing their chance to interact.
  - Invite them to join a game, like pool or cards, where the conversation can be focused on the game at first.

Because I didn't understand my course, I immediately hated every minute of work I had to do for it. But everything else to do with university, outside of the actual work, was fantastic. I was based in Liverpool, which is an awesome city, and I was living with a group of people I got on with straight away. God, meeting new people can sometimes be so awkward, can't it? Especially with the added pressure of knowing you've got to vaguely get on because you're now going to *live together*. The small talk that first week was painful. 'Where are you from?' ... 'Uh, okay I know someone from Sheffield ... Katie? Do you know her?' ... 'No ... Oh.' *silence* Yeah, awks. When one of my new flatmates informed us that he made his own wine though, I knew we'd be alright. Paul is still convinced to this day that his homebrew tasted okay. Sorry Paul, it didn't – it tasted like vinegar mixed with half a litre of vodka, neither of which had ever seen a grape in its life. Obviously, we all drank barrels of the stuff; it was a great ice-breaker.

I'm still friends with many of those same people now. (There's a story or two I could relate about the people that I'm not still friends with, but this isn't the time or place.) I'm incredibly lucky that I've always found it pretty easy to make friends. I can get on with anyone really, so for me, going to uni and making pals was never a problem. The problem I *did* have was in telling people what had happened and about my campaigning. I found it much easier to be open about it on social media than I did in person, with potential new mates. How do you talk to people you've literally just met about stuff going on behind the scenes? 'Nice to meet you. Yeah, I'm a suicide prevention campaigner because in January this year ... Fancy a pint?' Nope. I didn't want to bring the mood down by spilling all the shit I was going through, and I also didn't want it to be the first and then only thing I was known for, so I didn't say anything. My new flatmates only found out about any of it a week after freshers when they heard a Radio 1 Newsbeat interview I'd done about Sam, mental health and my petition – which was now at 100,000 signatures (yay). It must have been pretty weird to suddenly hear your flatmate on the radio talking about loads of heavy stuff he'd not acknowledged in any way before! They were super-supportive though, and have been ever since, immediately signing the petition and sharing it on their social media.

When I went home for Christmas that year, I told my mum that I loved everything about uni, except uni. I still *hated* my course and had only one lecturer that I liked. I thought the rest were a bunch of self-righteous, self-obsessed, unimaginably boring people whose inflated sense of self-importance can only be described as verging on having a God complex. They were the sort of people who could make any subject mind-numbingly dull by doing nothing more than simply talking about it. Their collective monotonous droning still echoes in my ears today. Basically, I didn't like them very much and I started to like what they were talking about even less. I will add a disclaimer here though: I know lots of people who really enjoyed my course. I didn't, it wasn't suited to me, or rather I wasn't suited to it, but please don't *not* become an engineer based upon this testimonial. Just make sure you really like maths. And I mean, *really* like maths.

The problem with me is: I'm stubborn. I wasn't going to quit because I'd had one bad semester. I made it my goal to get the degree almost as a point of principle: think you can drum me out by bombarding me with incomprehensible formulas? Think again! I was determined to get through the year and pass my exams. So there I was, struggling by day to understand how 'x' could possibly equal 3.2, and growing my social media presence and talking about mental health legislation by night. That is, when I wasn't out on the town swigging questionable homebrewed wine. To say I was busy would be an understatement.

Shockingly, my stubbornness paid off and I passed that first year. Well, admittedly I was given what's called a 'soft pass', or 'sympathetic pass', which is basically them saying: 'Bless you for trying. You were so close it would be rude not to let you back in (and besides, we want your nine grand again next year).' I was delighted – hey, I'd done a bit of maths and at least some of it must have been right! But, more importantly, at this point – around June 2019 – the petition had nearly two hundred thousand signatures! My social media had also grown considerably and it was only a matter of time before we'd hear from the bigwigs: the people in power that held the keys to the change we wanted to see. They couldn't ignore us for ever. Right?

HOW TO START YOUR OWN CAMPAIGN

STEP 1: WORK OUT WHAT YOU WANT TO CHANGE AND WHY

Decide on a goal that is both specific and tangible. For example, rather than just calling 'for better mental health support', which is really broad, instead campaign for 'the creation of a local support hub'.

Once you know what you want to change, learn everything you can about it. It's not enough to think it's important, you also need to understand why it hasn't happened before. What are the potential barriers and how can they be overcome? Also, welcome criticism – it will give you a heads-up on potential sticking points so you can fine-tune your counter-arguments. I've always said to the people around me, 'If you're not criticising my ideas you're not helping.' Delivered in the right way, criticism is the best sort of encouragement there is, helping you to create a watertight campaign.

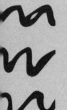

Identify who your decision makers are, anyone from politicians and CEOs to PAs. It's exceptionally important that what you're saying reaches the right ears. No matter how much support you get, if it doesn't end up in the right person's inbox, it's all for nothing (and also, no one will know who's meant to respond or what's meant to happen next).

STEP 2: DECIDE HOW YOU'RE GOING TO PRESENT YOUR IDEA

Presenting your idea effectively is absolutely crucial. It will enable you to drum up support and get noticed. Presentation can be in the form of a social media campaign, a petition, an open letter or a protest. Make sure whatever you end up doing though is targeted at the decision makers and is going to be seen/received by them.

STEP 3: PROMOTE YOUR IDEA AND CHASE EVERYONE FOR SUPPORT

Once you've decided how to present your idea and created a forum for it – promote it *everywhere*. Post about it on social media, send emails, put up posters, and find other activists in the same field who might be able to share or help.

While getting public support for your campaign is important, don't forget to personally chase the decision makers as well. Call their office, write letters, send emails, BE ANNOYING. There is a fine line between annoying and rude though. Don't be abusive, aggressive or insulting. Hold yourself to a high standard no matter how tempting it might be to lose your shit. It is possible to be both demanding and respectful. You've done a good job if the decision makers get sick of ignoring you and start engaging.

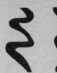

STEP 4: WORK THE MEDIA ANGLE LIKE A PRO

The media industry is like an aquarium where the big fish eat the small fish, so if you want to attract the biggies you must feed the small ones first. Instead of just contacting Sky News straight off the bat, contact your local paper or radio station. Campaigners can get quickly disheartened when major networks or media groups ignore their story, but that's not the way it works. I started out by approaching local news groups initially with my campaigns. My first media interview was a five-minute piece on BBC Radio Kent and one year later I was appearing on a live ITV show with an audience of over eight million. Feed the story to the small fish and watch the hungry big fish start circling.

(Sometimes the big fish do bite straight away though, so it is worth contacting them too. Just know that there is a process to this and it's likely you won't be on the front cover of the evening newspaper immediately – but that's not to say that you won't be eventually.)

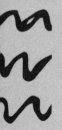

STEP 5: BE PATIENT

I'll be the first to admit that campaigning isn't easy. There's plenty of rejection and moments when it seems like nothing will ever change and you're shouting into the abyss. Have patience. Your decision maker can only ignore you for so long, especially if you continue to gain support and coverage. If things seem to be drying up then look into how you could present your idea differently. Could you organise a protest? Do you need a petition? Don't give up. Remind yourself why you're doing it.

STEP 6: SUCCESS! (HOPEFULLY)

This one's self-explanatory. Well fucking done – you're awesome.

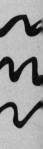

'WILL YOU SUPPORT MY PETITION, BORIS?'

My second year of university started and I found myself living in a tiny, overpriced student house with five other people, thinking Harry Potter didn't have it so bad in his cupboard under the stairs after all. I basically had to climb onto my bed if I wanted to close my bedroom door, and every morning without fail the next-door neighbour would go out for a fag, start coughing profusely and then vomit into his drain. It became my morning alarm. Another neighbour would get very drunk on her own and start either playing a vuvuzela or singing *really* badly with her dog trying to harmonise. But that's student life and I wouldn't have changed my house or housemates for the world. I loved it. (I still hated my course, but please refer to previous note re. stubbornness.)

That October, I was invited to the *Sun* newspaper's 'Who Cares Wins Awards', having been shortlisted for the Mental Health Hero Award. Two things struck me about this. First, this was my first award nomination and I found it a bit strange. While it was obviously an honour to be recognised for the hard work, and while the nomination confirmed that said work was making an impact (which was reassuring), I'd never done any of it to get a medal – I'd done it because it was necessary. The way I saw it, I wasn't doing anything special or outstanding because I shouldn't have to do it in the first place. The fact that

I did was the entire problem. This kind of campaigning shouldn't be rewarded but expected. If you'd seen what I'd seen and had the conversations that I'd had and then *not* done exactly what I'd done, that would have been more surprising to me than the fact that I was doing it. Second, Liverpool and the *Sun* have a famously terrible relationship and I felt pretty shady about attending an awards' ceremony from an institution despised by my host city. However, I figured that the possibility for some much-needed publicity about something I cared so passionately about trumped both of those concerns. Even if I didn't win, I could spread the word about the petition and potentially get legislation changed or updated. And I could also rinse the free bar.

I took Paul with me. Yes, he of the homebrewed wine. We arrived at the venue, went through security, had our suits patted down, our bags scanned, and travelled up to a conference floor of the London skyscraper where the ceremony was taking place. I remember clear as day Paul whispering to me, 'Ben, am I allowed to swear inside or do I have to sound posh?' as we mingled with the incredibly well-dressed attendees, nominees and celebrities. We helped ourselves to the complimentary prosecco and got the night started. When we were asked to take our seats for the formal dinner we scanned the name tags on our table: 'Kate Silverton, Jane Moore, Ben West ... The Rt Hon Boris Johnson MP'. Paul and I looked at each other, eyes wide and disbelieving. 'I'm meant to be sitting next to the prime minister,' I hissed. Yeah, that was unexpected. We topped ourselves up with prosecco and tried to collect ourselves, at which point one of the organisers came over and said: 'I'm not sure if you're aware, but the prime minister is attending tonight?' Er, yeah, I saw that. 'And he's requested to speak to you after the event,' she continued.

Erm, what now?

Why did I suddenly feel like I'd been told to go to the head-master's office at school? What on earth did the prime minister want with me? Oh well, another prosecco please.

We had dinner (minus the PM, much to my relief. When I'd first believed he was coming, I'd suddenly found it difficult to remember which way round you were meant to hold a knife and fork, and whether it was acceptable to dip a bread roll into your soup). Afterwards, the awards were announced – and I only went and won! I was genuinely surprised, but when I went to collect my award from Lorraine Kelly, I managed to pull together an off-the-cuff speech and look reasonably sober and presentable for the press photos. Around this time, the PM arrived with his army of staff, wandering through a – I'm going to be honest here – rather unexpected sea of adoring fans. He delivered a short speech celebrating the NHS (mentioning in particular how he'd overruled previous restrictions to intro-duce toasters back to the wards, describing the UK as an omelette and the NHS as the egg. Touché, and also, WTF?). A little later someone pulled me into a side room for a chat with him and I was very surprised to find an entire media produc-tion team with cameras hovering around two chairs. So much for a casual chat. I'd inadvertently found myself about to discuss seriously important stuff with Boris Johnson, the man who could actually get shit done, in front of a TV crew, while a bottle of prosecco down. Wonderful.

We shook hands and got some small talk underway. When it was clear this wasn't what the TV crew had in mind, I interrupted the PM mid-sentence, turned to the crew and said, 'Sorry, did you want us sitting down for this?' The audacity, Ben! Who did I think I was? Andrew Marr? Listen Boris, I'm the captain now. We sat down and started again, and about halfway through the conversation it properly hit me: *I was talking to the prime minister! The buck stops with him. This is as good as it gets as far as making waves is concerned. Forget small talk. I need to pin him down and get him on the record.*

'We've got this petition to the government that says we believe all teachers should be trained in mental health first aid as part of teacher training. Would you support that?' YES, BEN. Boris looked over his shoulder at his personal secretary, who sort of nodded, and he quickly said, 'Yes, the government would back that.' And, this is the important bit, he then said, 'It's vital.' I remember feeling like I'd just summited Everest – I'd got the PM to say *on camera* that my petition was vital. VITAL.

During the handshakes and goodbyes, I asked his private secretary, 'So, what happens next?', and was handed a flurry of business cards. Paul and I then returned to the main dining room to find some celebrities dancing and singing on a table and, while waiting for another prosecco, I sent an email to every single person who'd handed me their cards: 'It was so lovely meeting you all and please extend my thanks to the prime minister for our conversation. Do let me know the next steps for taking this further. Ben.'

And that, as they say, was a wrap.

DOWN TO DOWNING STREET

Paul and I travelled back to Liverpool the next day, arriving home in the evening, exhausted and more than a smidge hungover. As soon as we staggered through the door, my phone pinged and I opened a bizarre email: 'The prime minister would like to invite you to 10 Downing Street tomorrow to formally hand him the petition in person. Please arrive at 8 a.m.' Wait, what now? I was totally bewildered. *Downing Street? Eight a.m. tomorrow? Prime minister? Me?* But, but ... I'd just met him. And was already back in Liverpool. And ... did this mean the petition was going to be taken on? Did this mean it might become law? OH MY GOD. I HAD TO GO TO DOWNING STREET TOMORROW.

The email said I could invite four guests to go with me and that I'd need to submit all of their details to the Metropolitan Police so they could check we weren't going to kidnap the cat. I'd then need to write a letter, personally addressed to the PM, introducing the petition and laying out exactly what we were calling for. And – here was the big one – I'd need to deliver a *hardcopy of the petition.* Yes, I'd need to print out all 210,622 signatures (please feel free to flag up the sustainability concerns of printing out thousands of sheets of paper to Number 10 – they're definitely valid).

Where on earth do you print out 210,622 signatures, equating to *nine thousand* sheets of paper, in a matter of hours? My dodgy old printer certainly wasn't going to cut it. It was touch-and-go whether it could print out an essay. Also, I couldn't justify the sheer waste of paper, so I ended up reformatting the pages until I'd reduced the number to 281. Still not ideal – either environmentally or practically – but certainly better than the nine thousand it could have been. Could you imagine how unpopular I'd be if I'd tried to print that many thousands of pages out in the university library? Not to mention how much it would cost. I'd invited a few of the friends who'd been involved from the start, as well as my mum (who managed to print everything off for me last minute), to join me at Downing Street, apologising for the incredibly last-minute planning. I submitted all of their details to the Metropolitan Police and was relieved when they confirmed that none of them were terrorists, cat-nappers or had any outstanding arrest warrants. I wrote the letter to the PM, threw a few things into a bag and got back on a train to London that evening.

I find it hard to describe the feeling I had as I stood on the steps of 10 Downing Street, handing over a box of 210,622 signatures to the prime minister. And yes, I keep repeating the exact number because every single one of those people was there with me at that moment. I felt an immeasurable sense of pride as well as responsibility. I genuinely believed that box had the power to create change and that this was the start of something big. I was definitely pretty emotional. Look how far we'd come! Look at what we'd achieved! Who would have thought I'd be there? Not me, that's for sure. I felt like I could finally say I'd made Sam proud and I felt a bit of the guilt and the shame fall away.

It was a truly magical moment.

People have asked, 'So, what was Boris like?' and, I'll be honest, he surprised me. I expected some small talk, but not much else. However, he was very engaged with the topic, even out of sight of the cameras, and it felt genuine. He even discussed his own experiences with me. It felt like this meeting had more substance to it than to simply keep us happy and get a good story for the press. Especially when he had to be dragged away by a civil servant to attend another meeting. Afterwards, we were taken upstairs to 'The White Room' for tea and to talk to one of the education advisors about actually action-ing our petition, and that conversation *was* unremarkable. It seemed very much to me like she was on the defensive, constantly reiterating what they *were* doing and what they *were* delivering on. My insistence that whatever it was absolutely wasn't good enough definitely fell on deaf ears. But at the time I was so star-struck by the fact that I was sitting on the same sofa that Barack Obama had once sat on, it didn't really register. A tour of Number 10 followed, we took some snaps outside the infamous black door, I did a short interview for the Associated Press, and then we all had breakfast.

The response on social media was mad. I guess because it was as unexpected to everyone else as it was to me, the posts of us at Downing Street got everyone excited. We'd done it! *We* had done it. Together we had forced the most important office in the country to listen and, hopefully, to make changes. And, after that, everything seemed to go into overdrive. I found myself nominated and shortlisted for three other awards: Pride of Britain, JustGiving and the Diana Award. Of course, the recognition was greatly appreciated and proved what we were doing was working – that the message was getting out there and, more importantly, people were taking notice. Of particular pride to me was winning the Diana Award. That's something I really cherish. Every two years, 20 young people are selected from around the world and awarded a Diana Legacy Award in memory of Princess Diana. Diana was the epitome of a changemaker, never afraid to call for change or go against the status quo. She was the embodiment of empathy, morality and courage. Everyone will recognise the photos of her hugging the child with HIV, or visiting the minefields of Angola. The impact of her work is incalculable – she changed and saved many lives. She's always been a hero of mine and to be recognised as part of her legacy is truly the honour of my life. But, as much as it is an honour, it's also a responsibility. I have to continue, I can't give up. I can't stop educating or campaigning or protesting, because people depend on me doing so. That's a powerful perspective and one I take very seriously.

As part of that ceremony, I met HRH Prince William. I was more nervous about the correct way to address him and introduce myself than I was about what to say afterwards. Is it, 'Hello your highness' first, or, 'Hello your royal highness'? We'd been told all of that, but I couldn't remember it for the life of me. He didn't care though. He was such a normal guy and we had a really relaxed conversation. He came across as much more down-to-earth than many of the supposed 'celebrities' I'd met at other events. At one point he went over to Erick Venant, an antimicrobial resistance campaigner from Tanzania, and appeared to have a conversation with him in Swahili?! What a legend. You can quote me on that for his coronation. Maybe put it on his pound coins.

Phew! What a whirlwind. The end of 2019 was a mad, exciting and non-stop time. I felt on top of the world and everything was going so well . . . or so it seemed.

SCHOOLS VS MENTAL HEALTH: THE STORY SINCE 2018

In September 2020, the mental wellbeing teaching requirements were updated within the PSHE curriculum for both primary and secondary schools. These rules state that primary school students should learn:[11]

* that mental wellbeing is a normal part of daily life, in the same way as physical health;
* that there is a normal range of emotions (e.g. happiness, sadness, anger, fear, surprise, nervousness) and scale of emotions that all humans experience in relation to different experiences and situations;
* how to recognise and talk about their emotions, including having a varied vocabulary of words to use when talking about their own and others' feelings;
* how to judge whether what they are feeling and how they are behaving is appropriate and proportionate;
* the benefits of physical exercise, time outdoors, community participation, voluntary and service-based activity on mental wellbeing and happiness;
* simple self-care techniques, including the importance of rest, time spent with friends and family, and the benefits of hobbies and interests;

»

* that isolation and loneliness can affect children and that it is very important for children to discuss their feelings with an adult and seek support;
* that bullying (including cyberbullying) has a negative and often lasting impact on mental wellbeing;
* where and how to seek support (including recognising the triggers for seeking support), including whom in school they should speak to if they are worried about their own or someone else's mental wellbeing or ability to control their emotions (including issues arising online);
* that it is common for people to experience mental ill-health. For many people who do, the problems can be resolved if the right support is made available, especially if accessed early enough.

Meanwhile, secondary school students should learn:[12]

* how to talk about their emotions accurately and sensitively, using appropriate vocabulary;
* that happiness is linked to being connected to others;
* how to recognise the early signs of mental wellbeing concerns;
* common types of mental ill-health (e.g. anxiety and depression);
* how to critically evaluate when something they do or are involved in has a positive or negative effect on their own or others' mental health;

* the benefits and importance of physical exercise, time outdoors, community participation and voluntary and service-based activities on mental wellbeing and happiness.

Apart from the obvious fact that the primary school lesson objectives are clearly more accurate, useful and comprehensive than those detailed for secondary schools, this is actually really progressive and positive. Bearing in mind that when I started my petition in 2018 none of this was mandatory, things are moving in the right direction, and that makes me proud and hopeful. Who knows if any of it is directly linked to the petition, but it sure won't have hurt.

There's still much to be done though. PSHE lessons are only recommended for one hour a week and mental health is part of a rotating curriculum, meaning that, while teaching it at some point during the school year is required, schools also have to cover numerous other subjects within the same lesson, including relationships, health, and, in the case of secondary schools, sex education. It's also down to individual schools to decide the weighting of each subject, meaning they can choose to give more time to one than another.

WHAT ABOUT TEACHER TRAINING?

As of September 2021, teacher-training organisations are still under no statutory requirement to educate trainees about mental health. In other words, the government has made it mandatory that all

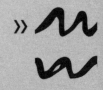

schools teach students about mental health – but hasn't made it mandatory that teachers are educated in how to teach it.

If the government thinks it's so important for students to be able to 'recognise the early signs of mental wellbeing concerns' then why doesn't it think the same is true for teachers? This is despite the prime minister telling me, to my face, that such education is 'vital'. It's also despite former Prime Minister Theresa May announcing in a press release on 17 June 2019[13] that it would be something her government would prioritise. It's been *years* and it's still not ingrained in law that all newly qualified teachers will be adequately prepared for the job they have to do.

So, once again – and I've lost count of the number of times I've said this – I call on the government to make mental health first aid a compulsory part of teacher training. Hell, I call on the prime minister personally: if you think this is truly 'vital', why hasn't it come up once since I spoke to you? Do you want to know how I know that nothing's changed? It's because I've spent the past three hours of my life reading the entire initial teacher-training criteria and supporting advice document, as well as the Education Regulations Law 2003, which outlines exactly what makes a teacher legally a teacher. No, it's not a fun read. No, I didn't enjoy reading it. But I enjoyed reading it far less when I learned that nothing has significantly changed since my call for action. I'm bloody tired, my eyes are hurting from looking at my screen, I can't be arsed to dress this up all nice and pretty, so let me make this as clear as I possibly can:

Dear Prime Minister: introduce a new statutory requirement for ITT (initial teacher training) that all trainee teachers will receive mental health first aid training.

What else do I have to do? Do you want a rap battle? Do you want to appear with me on a special episode of *Ru Paul's Drag Race UK*? Do you want me to dress up as the Education Regulations Law 2003 and dance around Parliament Square? Because I will. I'll do whatever it takes because that's how much I believe this is necessary and obvious. And let's not forget that hundreds of thousands of people agree with me.

Get. It. Done.

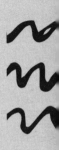

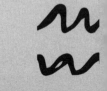

TAKEAWAYS

- Everyone can make a difference. You have a voice. Signing petitions, promoting causes you care about and pushing for things that matter really can trigger meaningful change.

- Don't drink a bottle of prosecco before meeting the prime minister.

- Meeting new people and/or attending events is intimidating for EVERYONE – yes, even Social Sally with her perfect line in rude jokes – so stop beating yourself up for it. Instead, name it to tame it.

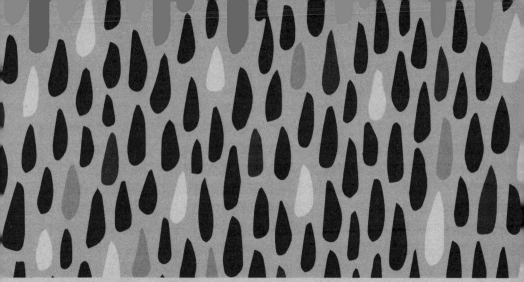

CHAPTER 6
BURNOUT

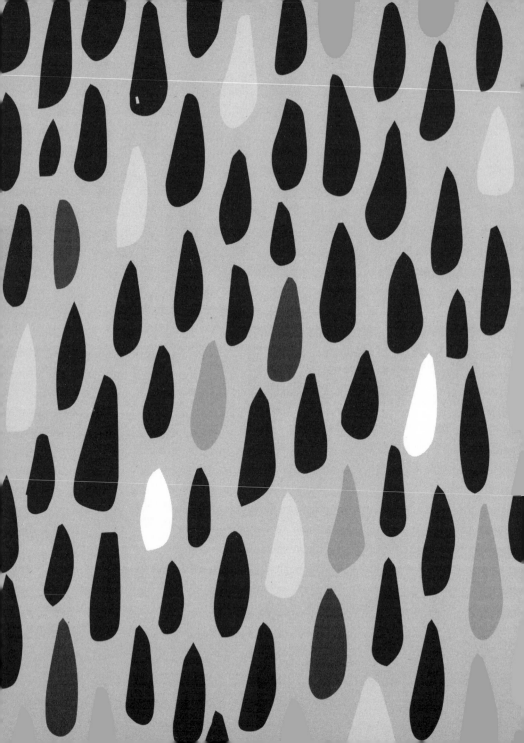

I'm writing this chapter sitting in my garden. Even though it's August, it's ridiculously cold, damp and windy, so I'm wearing a massive hoodie. The only noise I can hear, apart from the clacking of my keyboard, is the birds singing; it's very peaceful. Nature has always been something I've connected with. I guess growing up in the middle of nowhere, surrounded by trees and fields, will do that to you. The calmness of the woods was where I found solace immediately after Sam died. It was a place I went to feel part of something bigger than myself, and I found – and still find – it settling. Nature has become my happy place, an environment where I can slip into a state of calmness and freedom.

As a society, I feel that we've separated ourselves from nature, when, let's not kid ourselves, we *are* nature. We can pretend all we want that our tech and gadgets elevate us above a simpler life, but we are still very much connected to an older, wilder system. Our natural habitat isn't steel and concrete and our bodies aren't built to sit at a desk for eight hours a day or be sedentary (hence why reported back problems rocketed during lockdown[1]). We forget that, yes, while we may have adapted socially and mentally to live a 'modern life', our physiology is struggling to catch up. We've outperformed evolution because our 'prehistoric' brains are still wired to forage and live in the woods – and one of the biggest examples of this is the fight-or-flight response.

Fight or flight is your body's in-built threat detector; its way of trying to keep you safe by sensing potential danger. Back when we were living it large in the wild, inventing fire and painting the sides of caves, the main threats we encountered would have been physical (from animals or other cave-folk). There you'd be, sweeping up your cave and minding your own business, when suddenly you'd look up to find a leopard stalking the fire pit. The part of the brain that controls fear, known as the amygdala, would activate your hypothalamic–pituitary–adrenocortical axis (which is too many letters for any word), the response system that regulates hormones. This would then flood your body with cortisol and adrenaline, making your heart rate pick up, pumping blood away from the places that don't need it (including your digestive system, which is why you may feel nauseous, and also your fingers and toes, which is why you may literally experience 'cold feet' – that's where the expression comes from) to the muscles that do for either fighting or running. Blood vessels in your skin constrict to ward against excessive blood loss if the leopard takes a swipe at you, and you sweat more to stop from overheating, making you look pale and clammy. Your pupils dilate and hearing sharpens (allowing you to better see and hear the threat), you breathe more rapidly to oxygenate the blood, and even your sense of pain diminishes. Most importantly though, your rational and logical mind take a backseat (your brain knows you don't have time to think, 'Hmm . . . I wonder if it's already eaten today?'), leaving the action part in charge.

You are now a lean, mean fighting or running machine, ready to either lose a fight or a race with a leopard.

A ridiculous example, right? Who's bumping into leopards nowadays? Well, I am. A few years ago, I was fortunate enough to be invited out to South Africa to stay on a wildlife reserve. One day, my friends and I decided to cycle through a part of the reserve to check out the view from the top of a hill. 'What kind of idiot would *cycle* through a South African wildlife reserve?!' I hear you shout. THIS KIND *points thumb at self*. I managed to get ahead of the group and stopped to take in the breathtaking scenery. Looking up the path I then made eye contact with the most ENORMOUS leopard standing in the middle of the track. Given this is a book, you might expect a descriptive piece about the leopard – maybe some information on what kind it was, whether it had any scars, or – I don't know – its family set-up. Well, sorry to disappoint but the only thing I noticed was that it was *fucking huge*. I have no idea what I imagined a leopard looked like, but I certainly wasn't expecting an animal the size of a sofa. Pictures always make them look more like oversized, athletic tabby cats than something that could kill a person just by sitting on them.

I froze, still as a statue. A mosquito could have bitten every single millimetre of my arm and I wouldn't have flinched. Freezing is actually a key part of fight or flight – so much so that the whole rigmarole is also known as the fight, flight or freeze response – but it's much less talked about, which is an error because it happens *all the time*. Freezing usually occurs before fight or flight kicks in, when your body is assessing how much of a threat there is and what can be done about it. By staying still your body is limiting distractions while also making you less of a target. You know that comedy look of 'surprise' in cartoons: big eyes and wide-open mouth? That's spot-on. Your eyes get huge so you can see as much as possible, and your mouth prepares to either scream or take a big breath to aid running away. The next step is usually fight or flight, BUT, if you feel completely overpowered, trapped or can see no escape, your body can stay frozen (i.e. 'paralysed with fear'). This is why people can seem unresponsive in dangerous situations – their body is essentially 'playing dead' in the hope that the threat will go away or stop. When it is in that state, your brain can shut down the parts that process events so you don't form memories of what's happening, psychologically protecting you against trauma.

The next time a wasp interrupts a meal, check out everyone's various reactions: some people freeze and hope it goes away, some people flap and scream, and some just leg it and are never seen again – a perfect example of each aspect of this response.

So, there was me and the Dwayne Johnson of the leopard world having a stare-off and my brain was screaming: WOW, THIS IS HAPPENING. I'M GOING TO GET EATEN ALIVE AND ALL THE NEWSPAPER HEADLINES ARE GOING TO SAY: 'IDIOT BRIT MAULED TO DEATH WHILE CYCLING PAST LEOPARDS'. My rational brain had well and truly left the building (or, I should say, 'the reserve') and in that instant I couldn't for the life of me remember what I'd been told to do in such a situation: was I meant to leg it, stare it down, start screaming at the top of my lungs, throw my bike at it or make for the nearest tree? All I could think was: 'If I shout at it and I'm wrong, I'm fucked. If I stay still and I'm wrong, I'm also fucked.'

And then the leopard RAN UP A TREE. The bloody thing could *climb trees*! Who knew? Not me! That seriously put paid to Plan C, 'climb a tree', which would have clearly also left me fucked.

Anyway, it didn't eat me (thanks, Dwayne), but that situation is exactly what the fight, flight or freeze response has been designed for – to save you from life-or-death threats. However, we live in a world where the chance of a leopard attack is *really* slim (unless you're an idiot on a bike in the middle of a wildlife reserve), which is of course great news – but our bodies haven't caught onto that fact yet. Our bodies still think they need to prime us to either fight or run screaming into the trees whenever we feel threatened. We've been left with a pretty redundant system that cannot differentiate between 'threat' stress and 'general life' stress, meaning that your body may respond in exactly the same way upon receiving an overdue bill or a crappy WhatsApp message as it will upon facing a leopard. Not ideal.

Fight or flight is brilliant for short periods of danger, but feeling it *constantly* is very damaging, both physically and mentally. And in the modern world we experience it *all the time*. Exams, job interviews, dates, deadlines and so forth. Our bodies, though, aren't designed to be on 'high alert' 24/7.

AND . . . BURNOUT

As I explained at the end of Chapter 5, November 2019 was super-exciting and busy. Things were starting to happen and the work I was putting in was starting to make an impact. On the surface, everything appeared to be going really well. People who followed me on social media got used to seeing me at lots of events: collecting awards, meeting celebrities, chatting to the prime minister, generally looking like I was handling my shit and nailing life – but I wasn't. I've never really spoken to anyone about this, for reasons that we'll get into shortly, but behind the scenes, the end of 2019 was a very different story. I was stressed, I couldn't keep up with everything and, in short, I couldn't cope. I pushed myself so hard that I burnt out and had nothing left to give. In just a few weeks, I lost 10 per cent of my body weight, couldn't sleep at night, felt constantly unwell, had a persistent cold, and my body simply started to switch off. I've since discovered that these are common symptoms of burnout. Feeling that way and ignoring it only made everything worse. I wouldn't allow myself or my body to reset. I was hyper-aware that any lack of productivity would have to be made up for later and so I kept pushing harder to fill the gaps, filling my time with more and more and *more*.

University was increasingly unbearable – I couldn't do the work. I simply didn't understand it like everyone else did, so had to work doubly hard to complete the same assignment and then fail it anyway. And, outside of uni work, the campaigning was full-on. I'd be emailing or calling charities, organisations, universities, schools, politicians, government departments, having meetings, and doing interviews for podcasts, radio and TV. All of this meant travelling to and from Liverpool to London about twice a week. I'd get the train and then have to travel back, making it at least a six-hour round trip. I'd also be managing and trying to grow my social media accounts, a key tool in campaigning and connecting with people. Because of the Instagram algorithms, if you leave off posting or engaging for a while your posts don't get seen and you'll end up losing followers, so I had to keep up the momentum. Making good content takes time, especially when it's about such an important topic, so I'd have to create something, edit it, post it and then respond to the hundred or so responses I'd get . . . some of which were really distressing. The bigger my online profile grew, the more people would reach out and tell me that they were on the edge and ask for my help. If someone messages you, by name, to tell you something deeply personal that they haven't told anyone else, and they ask for your help, how are you meant to say no? I started getting invested. I felt a responsibility to help. And then one day, a follower told me they were worried about someone they knew who was suicidal. They asked what they should do – I gave them the details of support centres and the like, and said I was there for them . . . and then their friend died. They took their own life and I was blown away by it. I felt like I'd failed them. But I couldn't *not answer* those messages, could I? Especially not when I'd deliberately put myself in a position where I could help people. I'd actively sought it out. How could I then say, 'Nah. Too much, lads. I'm off?' I had gone into all of this because I wanted to help people, and so now, if I was asked to do a podcast or something that might help just one person, I didn't feel like I could say no. But that meant I didn't say no *to anything*. It became impossible to draw a line. I had a responsibility . . . but it was also becoming a burden, and I didn't want it to be. I just didn't know how to manage it well enough so that everything could work together.

And on it went: engineering, mental health, social media, family, friends, campaigning, travelling . . . Then a bit more engineering, social media again, and then finally, a night out with my mates. Then a hangover the next day, which meant falling even further behind with uni work, so I'd prioritise that . . . Then I'd miss a campaigning meeting or deadline and then I'd look at my social media DMs and see hundreds there . . .

We went to London as a family one evening in December. It must have been about 5 p.m., so it was packed as we got onto the Tube, and Mum, standing next to me, looked at me and said, 'You look so tired.' Feeling defensive, I ignored her. But she was right. I was exhausted. Physically and mentally. I had little left to give. I look back on photos from that time and I can't help but notice how unwell I look: thin, pale and drained. Even when I'm smiling and having a good time, the effect everything was having was literally written on my body.

I had to keep going though. I didn't want to, make no mistake. Every day I wanted to drop out of uni and give them the middle finger as I left. Every day I wanted to say no to at least some of my other obligations, to come up for air. Even when I wasn't working, I'd lie in bed and my head would be spinning thinking about how planes fly, or Instagram algorithms, or what to say to that guy who hadn't left his room for four days. It consumed me. I had fallen victim, like so many millions of other people, to toxic productivity.

IF WE DON'T HAVE THE TOOLS TO DO THE JOB, WE ARE DESTINED TO FAIL.

TOXIC PRODUCTIVITY × MORAL RESPONSIBILITY = CRASH AND BURN

Toxic productivity affects almost all of us. It's a societal and cultural narrative that, depending on where you live, you've probably been taught your whole life. It's the belief that success (and 'worthiness') is found in constant *doing* – constant producing and achieving – and that if you want to be successful or 'good' you've got to work hard. And if you're not working hard enough you're letting yourself and everyone else down.

Toxic productivity is the expectation that you'll work overtime as a matter of course, with your boss or colleagues sending emails at 7 a.m. or 10 p.m. and expecting you to answer (or, if they don't, expecting you to at least acknowledge how hard *they're* working). It's the 'successpreneurs' posting selfies in the gym at 5 a.m. and advocating the philosophy that if you're not multitasking you're WASTING TIME. It's the feeling of guilt for watching TV, for taking time off, for having a break.

To an extent, yes, you need to work to achieve things. Nothing happens if you don't do anything. But at the same time, working for the sake of working or feeling guilty for not working hard enough is unnecessary. Working 12-hour days looks great on paper – 'Yay, I'm nailing this working hard lark!' – but in reality that isn't sustainable and you're actually probably not producing your best work (because you're knackered).

It's certainly nothing to be proud of (ever heard of a little thing called work/life balance?).

It comes back to my previous points about the exam-focused results culture in our schools. We cannot lay that amount of pressure on young people and not also educate them about stress. Imagine that you were never taught how to read and then were suddenly handed a Charles Dickens novel and told to analyse it. That's what we're doing when it comes to ignoring mental health education and then expecting kids to sit GCSEs and A-Levels and be able to cope with the pressure. If we don't have the tools to do the job, we are destined to fail. It's exactly this lack of understanding around anxiety, stress and fear that creates such high levels of burnout in the working world – and I have no doubt that not being taught about stress is what led to me falling apart in November 2019.

I was living under the impression that giving up any opportunities was bad. That if I wasn't working I wasn't doing enough, and that I could always work harder. I remember feeling so guilty when I wasn't doing something productive – say, if I was just watching Netflix – that I wouldn't even enjoy the show. And I was only 19 years old. I also didn't want to offend people. It's part of my nature that I want people to like me, and I think it's polite to say yes and to give them my time. It's easy to see now that I was pushing things too hard, but I couldn't bear to admit that to myself at the time because I felt that if I stopped working I would have failed and I couldn't let people see me as a failure.

So I worked myself to the point that I was ill.

I was almost exclusively in a state of fight or flight by November. My daily stresses became interpreted as dangers that would literally make my body shake. I'd not be able to eat or sleep, and I'd throw up thinking about uni deadlines, or punch my chair and break it. I had reached the point of burnout, which, according to the NHS, is 'a state of emotional, physical and mental exhaustion caused by excessive and prolonged stress. It occurs when an individual feels overwhelmed, emotionally drained and unable to meet constant demands.'[2]

This is the first time I've really thought back to that and analysed what was going on, and I'm only now realising how unwell I was. I was suffering from burnout, but the fact I couldn't work because I was ill made me even more stressed. Talk about a vicious circle.

Burnout is actually really common. According to a study by Asana, more than 70 per cent of workers say they experienced burnout in 2020.[3] The good news is that companies are taking notice, with LinkedIn giving its workers a paid week off in mid-2020 purely to de-stress, followed by the Nike management in Oregon announcing it was doing the same later that year. Best of all though, Scotland recently revealed it will be trialling a four-day working week.[4]

TAKING STOCK AND MAKING TIME

I realised after that trip to London with my family in December 2019 that I was in fact really struggling. I recognised that I had too much going on, which I guess was a good start, but I still felt like I had to keep the work up and the impression I was doing well. And, on paper, I wasn't actually doing badly – I was passing assignments and getting good grades . . . but at huge personal cost.

I made a pact with myself: I was going to have to change something to feel better. I took stock and realised that the time and stress demanded by many of the things I'd signed up for wasn't balanced out by the value gained. I had to be more selective with what I took on – I had to learn how to say 'no'. It's such a simple thing, isn't it, saying no? Yet, in practice, I find it near-enough impossible to do: 'What if I sound rude?' 'What if I sound unappreciative?' 'What if I lose the chance of a lifetime?' So, when it came to university, campaigning and extracurricular work, I devised a not-so-revolutionary way of solving the problem – a traffic-light system for my calendar:

- GREEN: Something of exceptional importance that cannot be missed. Not taking part in this could risk the failure of one of my goals.
- AMBER: Something with great potential, but that's not essential, so, *if time allows*, I can consider it.
- RED: Something that will have relatively little impact compared to other things – the cost in time is larger than the return value – so, even if I'd like to do it, THIS IS A NO.

Suddenly, I had a way of identifying what I could cut out in order to continue being able to ... well ... function. It gave me a level of control and also flexibility, and, most importantly, a clear view of what I HAD to turn down or cancel. I won't lie, it didn't change my life overnight and I would still end up struggling to get everything done, but it was the start of me recognising that I couldn't and shouldn't do everything. That I had to look after myself.

On which note, I also added time-outs into my schedule: actual booked-in no-work zones. I've always really struggled to switch off in down-time, so, by scheduling it in, I could accept it because it was 'official'. Obviously, there's a deeper problem there that I needed to look into (as to why I thought breaks were unproductive), but at the time this worked as a temporary measure in enabling me to switch off sometimes. And I soon learned that time away from work and regular breaks make you much more productive than just constantly slogging away – which is the entire argument behind the four-day work week: people get more work done in four days than five because they're refreshed, revitalised and less resentful. They're also working to the time schedule they have, rather than exhaustedly dragging stuff out. It just goes to show the power of down-time and how much stress affects our day-to-day productivity.

Social media had to change for me too, especially after I nearly spat out my drink analysing my 'screen time' data and saw how much of my life I'd given over to online. I set myself some rules:

- Don't post drunk. It had happened before and I'd wake up in the morning to 10 missed calls and 20 texts telling me to delete something that *definitely* should not be public.
- Limit the time I spend on social media to doing only what I needed to do, i.e. posting stuff and interacting with people. *Not* mindlessly scrolling through reams of nonsense.
- Limit who I followed to those who checked at least one of the following criteria:
  Do they entertain me?
  Do they educate me?
  Do they inspire me?

I ended up unfollowing so many people on Instagram that my account was actually suspended. Oops (worth it though). Too often we follow people who make us feel shit, even if we know them or like them. For me, my social media used to be filled with those who amplified that toxic productivity narrative and made me feel guilty for having a break. I got rid of them all. (If you don't feel you can unfollow someone for whatever reason – i.e. it's your friend but their posts make you feel rubbish – you can always simply 'mute' them instead. You won't see anything they post and they won't know they've been muted so won't be offended. Win-win.)

Some other tricks to consider that I didn't implement, but that might help:

- Remove the social media apps from your phone (without disabling your accounts) so you don't look at them on autopilot. You can still log on via the website, but it'll be a choice rather than mindless clicking.

- If WhatsApp is getting you down, you can turn off the blue tick notifications (which will remove them both for you and other people) and also the 'last seen' information. This relieves the pressure of feeling you have to respond and wondering why other people haven't.

- If you want a quick break from all your apps, but don't feel the need to delete them from your phone, go to your 'mobile data' settings and deselect them so they won't work on 3G or 4G, and then turn off your Wi-Fi. The apps will only update again when you reselect them to work with mobile data and/or when you turn on your Wi-Fi.

HOW TO SAY NO POLITELY BUT FIRMLY, WITHOUT OFFENDING ANYONE

Honestly, it's worth offending people to protect your own health sometimes. Everyone has different 'rules' regarding social acceptability and 'selfishness', but one person's definition of rude is another person's definition of self-care. You can look after yourself without being obnoxious and hurting other people's feelings, but remember: being selfish isn't always a bad thing. I wish I'd offended a lot more people, because I would have felt a lot better. Obviously this is much easier said than done though, so here are some things I've said in the past to politely but firmly dodge events:

* 'I'm so sorry, I've actually double-booked myself. I'm going to have to give it a miss this time, but hopefully we can reschedule.'
* 'Being fully transparent, I honestly can't take anything more on at the moment. I hope you can understand. Maybe next time.'
* 'Sorry, I'm actually just having a chilled one tonight.'

Honesty is often the best policy here, so you don't have to keep track of excuses.

My burnout taught me that we really need to listen to our bodies more. Human brains know what they're doing, so if they're screaming at you to STOP, you need to stop. You shouldn't feel guilty about rewatching *Peep Show* for the fifteenth time that afternoon in bed with a cup of tea and a tub of ice-cream if that's what you need! And we all need that sometimes. For me that also means allowing myself time out in nature, being among the birds and trees, going for a run, looking after my plants, lying on the floor with a dog (any dog). Most importantly, it's about recognising when I need to take that time – the act of stopping is great, but the realisation that you need to is the biggest step. Checking in with myself is the biggest thing I've learned about looking after my own mental health:

'How are you doing, Ben?'
'Not bad, thanks Ben.'
'Sound – crack on then, mate.'

Deciding to prioritise your mental and physical health can feel like a big decision. It can be easy when you're young to think you have to throw yourself at every opportunity that comes your way so as to get the chance to be successful. I did exactly that because I couldn't bear the thought of letting anyone down or feeling like a failure. So, even though I'd started putting boundaries in place – and even though they were working – I knew there was one HUGE thing hanging over my head. One colossal decision that would change everything . . .

I had to leave university.

SEE YOU LATER, AEROSPACE ENGINEERING

I was terrified of making the call to actually leave my university course. What was everyone going to think and how would I ever get a job? I'd been taught that the only path to success was via university: you get a degree and then you get a job. So, even though I couldn't stand my degree course, I plodded on. But now, I had to get out. It was just a case of when and how.

The final straw for me came in my third year during my dissertation. Yes, I'd made it two and a half years into a three-year course. And, I'd thought I was onto a winner with my dissertation because I'd partnered up with somebody brilliant; for ease I'm going to call him George. He'd actually *chosen* to work with me, saying I came across as switched on and like I knew my shit. Ha! Was I going to tell him the truth? Of course not! I remember being on the phone to my mum and saying, 'It's fine, I've got some engineering god as a partner, so it'll be okay.' It was not okay. The theme of my dissertation was: 'Design and build a multi-use remote-piloted aircraft that can carry modular payloads and undertake functions such as cartography, crop analysis and delivering foreign aid.' Fuck. I don't even know where to start with that. I was mere months away from graduating and I still didn't really understand how planes fly.

One winter evening in 2019, I was on the phone to George when he asked me to calculate the tail volume coefficient of our plane. 'Oh yeah, sure thing,' I replied. 'Can't wait. Shall we call back in an hour to discuss?' I know as much as you do about tail volume coefficients – which is nothing at all. But of course I wasn't going to tell him that. I had to keep up this act that I knew what I was doing.

The panic that set in as soon as I hung up the phone cannot be adequately expressed here – I immediately emailed someone on my course, told them I was leaving, and then texted George very apologetically telling him I'd spontaneously quit university. Surprise!

As it turns out, calculating the tail volume coefficient really isn't that difficult. A simple google brings up the formula. But I didn't drop out because of that – quitting was two and a half years in the making. Two and a half years of hating my course and struggling with it. So sending that email delivered the greatest sense of relief I have ever experienced and the following few days were magical. I instantly felt more energised and happier. I still had the voice in the back of my mind going, 'Well, you've fucked it. What on earth are you going to do now?' But right then those thoughts were drowned out by literally every other part of my body singing with joy that it had finally ended.

University is not for everyone. And I'm not just saying that. There is no shame in realising it's not for you and leaving. I actually wish I'd left sooner. I wouldn't have changed who I met, or any of the experiences I had outside of my course, but everything other than that – no thanks. If you get second thoughts about your course, or feel like you're burning out and your lecturers don't give a toss, then don't feel cowed about demanding what you're paying for. You're spending a lot of money to attend, so you can throw your weight around a bit. Next, really think about why you're still there and what you want to get out of it. Can you get that somewhere else? On another course? At another institution? Perhaps you can secure more support, some extra help, or can defer for a year. But don't forget, there are a lot of other great options out there – other life paths just as valid and exciting that can be explored via vocational courses, apprenticeships and work experience. I know a lot of people feel the same pressure I did to stick with it. There is an enormous amount of societal expectation surrounding higher education, but here are some of the things that I achieved outside of it:

- I became a non-executive board member for a multinational brand advising on long-term brand strategy.
- I was involved in meetings with government departments advising Westminster on policies regarding education and health.
- I wrote a book (oi oi).
- I am starting out in a career that means a lot to me and that I find real value in. I enjoy what I do and it feels meaningful.
- I haven't endangered any lives by being allowed to design planes that real people will travel on that would certainly crash because they wouldn't be able to fly, ever.

I am not saying any of this to brag. In fact, I would encourage all of you to make a list of your achievements if you feel like you're struggling right now – things that you're proud of having done or got through. Too often, especially in our self-deprecating culture, we mistake pride for vanity. I have written the above list because I was very much given the impression that I might be throwing away my professional future by dropping out of university. And yet, so far, so good. (To be clear, I'm not saying that everyone should jack in higher education. I'm saying that often we do things because we feel we *should* without ever considering whether it's right for us. You do have a choice.)

University in general, and my personal experience of it, features large in Chapter 7 when I discuss lockdown, so I won't go into more detail now, but suffice to say that finally making that decision to leave my course helped enormously to alleviate the symptoms of burnout. I'd been like a duck before, looking all serene and chilled on the surface while its legs paddled madly underneath. Leaving uni gave me the space to breathe, reassess and reset. To focus on myself and my campaigning. To acknowledge that actually things hadn't been manageable: it wasn't a case of me failing or not being up to the task; what I'd been asking of myself was ridiculous. And yes, now I had to forge a path without the backup of a degree (which I'd been constantly told was my golden ticket to a successful career), but the difference in my physical and mental health, once I finally decided to make changes to prioritise them, was so noticeable that I knew I'd done the right thing. Of course, I didn't realise this overnight. I was never going to wake up one morning and, midway through brushing my teeth, be like, 'Wow! I feel fucking fantastic – good job, Ben!' Rather, it was a process of learning and adapting, with the really simple goal of looking after the person in the mirror just that little bit more than I'd done the day before.

NOT ALL STRESS IS BAD

Stress works on a spectrum. On one end you have zero stress (think sunbathing in the Caribbean) when your cortisol levels will be extremely low. On the other end of the spectrum, when you're significantly stressed (think boss calling you into a meeting to discuss 'your behaviour at last night's Christmas party') your

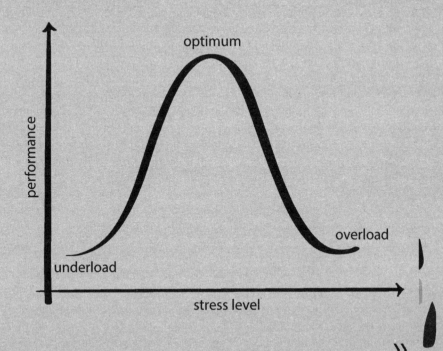

»

cortisol levels will have rocketed and you'll be in fight-or-flight mode. However, there is a middle zone – an optimum position – where the levels of cortisol increase your complex cognitive function. In layman's terms, this means that your brain is working more effectively and you're actually functioning on top form.

Having no stress at all isn't actually good for us. It means we underperform. Yet equally, having too much stress isn't ideal either. Once our cortisol levels rise above the optimum level, our complex cognitive function becomes less effective as our body starts to interpret the external world as dangerous and it goes into fight-or-flight mode, reducing our productivity and performance. The trick is learning to recognise when you're tipping over into the fight-or-flight danger zone and then working to calm your body down:

* Are you shaking or trembling?
* Does your body feel tense?
* Is your heart racing?
* Are you breathing faster or harder?
* Do you feel nauseous?
* Are your pupils dilated?
* Do you have cold hands or feet?
* Are you pale and clammy?

If so, read on . . .

HOW TO CALM YOUR BODY DOWN

Regain control of your breathing:

* Find a place that is quiet, safe and away from distractions.
* Sit comfortably or lie down on the floor.
* Inhale slowly and deeply over a count of eight seconds and feel your stomach expanding outwards.
* Hold the breath for a count of eight seconds before slowly releasing it, again for another eight-second count.
* Repeat this for a minute or until you start to feel calmer.

Yoga is brilliant at calming you down when in a heightened state. It does this by bringing your attention back to the present moment, to your body, and so away from fears and stresses. There are free online yoga videos you can check out, with routines lasting anything from 10 minutes to an hour.

You can also reassure yourself with mantras or by rationalising the threat. In other words, by telling yourself that you're safe. It's important to say it in an appreciative way. So not: 'Oh come on, don't be ridiculous. It's only ___.' Rather: 'Okay, thanks for stepping in and for trying to help me, but I'm not in danger here and I'm safe.'

TAKEAWAYS

- Your health is more important than grades, work, socialising, social media and keeping other people happy. Look after it and don't feel bad about prioritising yourself.

- Burnout is a very real risk for everybody. Check in with how you feel physically, as the physical manifestations of stress are often the most obvious.

- Managing your commitments and learning how to say no is a key part of keeping a healthy balance within your life. If you're overwhelmed, start putting in place boundaries that will help you to work out what is essential, what's not, and what makes you feel both good and bad.

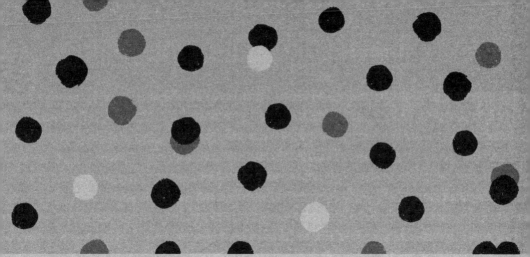

CHAPTER 7
ALL IN THE NAME OF ACADEMIC EXCELLENCE

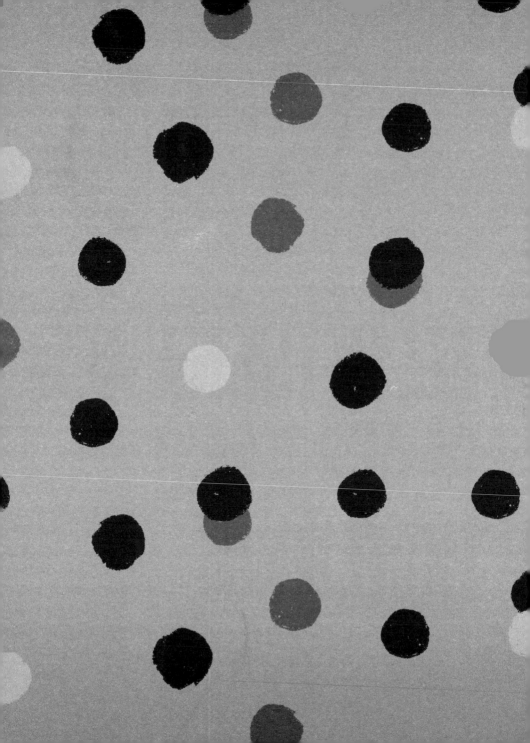

We talk a lot about tuition fees: debating value, inequality, inaccessibility, classism, privilege, debt, burden – the list goes on. So how much is it fair to expect to pay for a degree or a higher education qualification? Three thousand pounds per year? Ten? Twenty? How about one student's life? How about a hundred student lives? According to government data, between 2010 and 2019 a total of 1,324 students over the age of 18 died by suicide while studying in higher education. That means on average 132 students per year lose their lives to suicide.[1]

Student mental illness and suicide is something universities seem reluctant to address. For example, in 2020, an investigation into UCL's mental health support found services under-resourced, underfunded and understaffed.[2] And in 2021, the University of Edinburgh admitted to failing to provide adequate support to a student who died by suicide, despite there being numerous opportunities for intervention.[3] Mental health is not a snappy soundbite for a marketing campaign, not a pretty poster to pin up around campus, not a compassionless email sent to students as a box-ticking exercise. It is the student alone in their university accommodation purposefully taking an overdose; it's the student so overwhelmed by stress that they step in front of a train; it's the student who opens their friend's bedroom door to find them dead. Those three examples are real stories told to me by loved ones left behind. Student suicide is one of the most important issues our country faces today and we need to see it for what it really is – something that is preventable. Yes, some people will still take their own lives when they see no other option regardless of the support they receive. However, *some might not*. Surely we owe it to our young people to offer them that chance? Too often we see leaders talk the talk but never walk the walk, waiting for people to forget and move on. And, dutifully, we do just that.

You can probably sense my frustration and anger. That's because this, like so much else to do with the subject, is personal. I had the weird 'privilege' of experiencing university both before and during the Covid-19 pandemic. In September 2020, three months before I quit and a mere few weeks before university students were scheduled to return and begin the next academic year, we were still patiently waiting to hear how, or if, university would start again. The summer of that year had been relatively 'normal', with restrictions easing and people hoping the end of the crisis was in sight. I was convinced that the government would announce that all teaching would be moved online, encouraging people to stay at home in order to continue the positive direction the country seemed to be moving in with regards to the pandemic. Given that, at this point, no one was vaccinated and having in-person classes would mean roughly 2.5 million[4] people travelling around the country, it seemed pretty obvious that in-person teaching wasn't a great idea. In fact the government's own scientific advisors warned that Covid outbreaks were 'very likely in universities'.[5] Alas, the bigwigs decided that unis should remain open, with face-to-face teaching to be encouraged. Lectures were on! Classes were on! Group hugs all round.

I couldn't get my head around it. We seemed to be teetering on the precipice of things getting worse rather than better –

why take the risk? (This was at the time when it was still illegal to meet more than five of your mates at once and getting on public transport wasn't advised.) I had no choice though but to drive from my home in Kent all the way to Liverpool to start my third year. Because I had been weighing up quitting anyway, I hadn't signed up for any accommodation, but had found a small flat in the city centre. As someone living alone, I was allowed to have a social bubble with one other household, so I went to visit my friends the night I arrived. The day afterwards, I was informed I'd have to isolate for two weeks as I'd been in close contact with someone who had the virus. Yay. I'd made it the whole year without coming into contact with anyone with Covid yet achieved just one single day at university. And, that same week, the university saw the folly of the situation and informed us that all in-person teaching was going to be cancelled. Who'd have thought it, eh? Oh yeah. That's right: EVERYONE.

At first isolation was a novelty; an excuse to lie in bed all day watching Netflix. I told the critical voice in the back of my mind that no, I wasn't being lazy, I was *doing* isolation, and that worked for a bit. After a couple of days, however, isolation sucked. The aloneness became overwhelming. I'm a people person, I enjoy being around others. Now, suddenly I was going entire days without any contact at all and sometimes without even speaking out loud. I remember realising one day, at about 9 p.m., that I hadn't said anything all day and so made this little squeaking noise, then said, 'Well, this is really shit,' and turned back to Netflix. I was so bored I started pacing up and down my flat like a lion trapped in a zoo enclosure. The pacing eventually turned into jogging and I managed to complete 5 kilometres (yes, I felt sorry for whoever lived below me, but not sorry enough to stop).

Luckily for me, during my isolation I had friends to call and messages to respond to. I also knew others who were isolating, so we could commiserate together. I distinctly remember thinking: 'Imagine if I didn't know anyone. Imagine if I'd never lived away from home before. Imagine if I was anxious about starting uni on top of already being anxious about lockdown.'

There isn't a shadow of doubt in my mind that the decision to send university and higher education students back in September 2020 cost lives and caused suffering to many. Realistically, the mass incarceration of students within their accommodation was inevitable – *inevitable*. If *I* could see that happening – someone with no additional insight into Covid data – how the hell did those supposedly 'in the know' turn out to know fuck all? Two and a half million students found themselves at the mercy of government and university leadership that didn't have a plan, didn't know what they were doing, and then had to scramble to rectify a situation that never should have happened in the first place.

Since that time, higher education institutions have repeatedly told us that online teaching is just as good as in-person teaching and that it doesn't affect a student's ability to learn. On that basis, most, if not all, universities have refused to issue tuition fee refunds. However, if that is indeed the case, why were the higher-ups so determined to bring students back in September 2020, regardless of the risk?

My conclusion is simple: at no point did anyone seriously consider the effect on students' mental health. At my university, we used to get 'Covid-19 update' emails, informing us about any changes to the rules. Right at the very end, after multiple paragraphs detailing public health advice and the uni's commitment to their students' safety, was a sentence saying: 'We would like to remind you that our University Support Services are on hand if you need any additional support now or in the future.' Thanks, so helpful. Mental health hadn't been considered in the run-up to this shitshow, and now it was reduced to a postscript on an impersonal email.

Throughout the pandemic, the UK population had been told that it would need to make sacrifices to protect the vulnerable. And most people consistently did their best to protect the elderly, those with underlying health issues and those identified as more at risk. However, it is my opinion that an entire group of vulnerable people were overlooked: students. Young people who were forced to move away from their support network and then required to quarantine and isolate with strangers. They had to deal with a lot of very adult shit, alone, during an unprecedented time.

Why were they sent back? Perhaps because it had been ingrained in the cultural psyche by then that young people were more resilient to the illness – and that belief in physical resilience translated into a blanket belief about young people's resilience in general, including their mental stoicism. It could be something to do with the financial implications of students not moving into their halls. Perhaps it was also part of the urgency to 'get things back to normal', or maybe the folks in charge genuinely did believe that universities could deliver face-to-face teaching and offer students a positive experience. May I suggest, though, that the problem isn't found in what they *did* think about, but rather in what they clearly didn't.

A DEATH AND A RAGE

In October 2020 my worst fears were realised when news broke that a 19-year-old student named Finn had taken his own life in his halls of residence at a major university after experiencing severe anxiety during lockdown. I'm usually good at managing difficult conversations, having learned how to compartmentalise in order to protect myself. But this news hit me hard. I couldn't stop thinking about how awful it must be to feel that desperate – and utterly alone. How could this have been allowed to happen again? The familiar feeling of injustice bubbled up and became rage – pure red-hot rage. I was thrust back into the grief and anger I'd felt straight after Sam's death. Up until this point, I'd been doing a bit better. I'd been working through a lot with my (new) counsellor and had been making progress. But sometimes it felt like litter-picking in a landfill, and this news brought it all back. I had to say something so I propped my phone up onto my kitchen counter and pressed record. What poured out were thoughts from a brain gripped in the talons of grief. I did one take and uploaded it to Instagram. Opposite is an abridged transcript from that video:

I don't know if anyone's going to actually listen to what I'm about to say and I don't really care, I'm going to say it anyway. We are getting it wrong. Because if this is a suicide, watch the reaction from the University of Manchester: what they'll do is tell you everything they've done right. And anyone who reacts to an incident where someone has died by saying, 'This is what we've done right', is getting it fatally wrong. We need to get to a point where we can spot that we all have a role to play in preventing these deaths. We all have a role to play in finding it in ourselves to go, 'Right, I know I might be doing something, but what more can I do?' Because we cannot live in a world – and I cannot stress this enough – we cannot live in a world where we accept the fact that young people die because of their mental health. I'm sorry, we can't accept that and I'm not going to accept that. I'm getting so emotional about this because it's happening all the time and lots of people at university at the moment are stuck on their own and they are facing some demons. And we live in a society where it's okay to lose people, young people, to suicide. It's okay – it's just something in the statistics every year – and it makes me sick. One suicide for a young person is devastating. It is a failure of a system, it is a failure of a government, it is a failure of a university, it is a failure of society.

I cannot imagine for a second the pain that you have to endure to purposely inflict fatal injuries on yourself. That we accept that it happens is disgusting and it shows so much about our leadership in this country. It shows so much that we were sent back to university this year, it shows so much that the mental health of the student population was totally and blatantly ignored when we were told we had to return to university – return to jail cells, return to isolation, return to be separated from our families, separated from our friends. Thrown into a city that, for many, they'd never been to before, and sent there to be isolated and have our mental health totally ignored.

Our government is failing at the mental health crisis, they are failing and it's going to get worse before it's going to get better. We need change, we need empathy, we need humanity, and we have none of it with this government. We have none of it with this current leadership and I am sick of it because when I spoke to Boris Johnson, when I spoke to Theresa May, when I spoke to Esther McVey – when I spoke to these politicians they made it very clear to me that it is a priority to them to fix this issue. And yet they accept that the number of young suicides is not zero. They'll put money towards reducing that number, but they're ready to accept that there will be a number.

It makes me sick to think that this is another person that's lost their life to this. It makes me sick to think that we're going to have to see this many, many times again in the future. And I don't know if anyone's going to hear that, I don't know if anyone's going to listen to what I've just said. They don't see the people behind the numbers. They don't see a 19-year-old boy who spent a week in his room on his own, didn't speak to anyone, and ended up taking his own life. By sending us back to university, that is an admission of them being ready to accept that there will be students who kill themselves, and that it's worth it. It's not, and that lack of empathy and humanity in our leadership is sickening when it comes to mental health.

It. Is. Sickening.

As it turns out, people did listen – nearly nine hundred thousand people. The video was shared over and over again, far and wide, triggering an outpouring of stories from people reporting their own experiences of lockdown and mental illness at university. I was shocked by how far and how deep this went. People told me how their uni delivered boxes of mouldy food to halls while they were isolating. Others how their uni had sent police officers into their accommodation in the early hours of the morning, waking everyone up and threatening arrests and fines because they'd had dinner together as a floor. I was sent photos and videos of terrified students discovering they were being *fenced* into their accommodation with the fences patrolled by guards. They pleaded with me to do something to help because they believed they'd been physically locked in – the university had never contacted them to explain about the fences, they just appeared. That particular university later apologised for its lapse in judgement, but only after the students loudly and actively complained. And they complained because they were *frightened*. That instinctive reaction to being put in a cage of lashing out shows just how much these decisions were messing with people's mental health.

I started researching what I could do to try to help. What one thing could I champion that might make a serious tangible difference? It was written in the government guidelines that students in lockdown were allowed to leave and go somewhere else – e.g. back home, to a friend's or to hospital – if they believed they were in 'danger of harm'. That danger could be from someone else or from themselves. But not enough people knew this. Lots of students were continuing to isolate even though their mental health was deteriorating fast because they'd very much been given the impression that they couldn't leave. 'If you are struggling with your mental health at uni, you are allowed to break lockdown and go somewhere that is safer for you' was the message I repeated over and over again on all my social channels and in my DMs – anywhere I could. But I knew that, while this was integral for students to know, it wouldn't change the fundamental systemic issues that had got us into the situation in the first place, so that's where I turned my attention next.

THE MENTAL HEALTH UNIVERSITY LEAGUE TABLE

In December 2020, I dropped out of university (as I described in Chapter 6) – yay, no more maths! – but stayed on living in Liverpool, filling up notebooks with ideas and research. These ideas were then developed on a white board I'd put up in my room, which in turn spilled over into Post-It Notes stuck all over my walls and even my mirror. It was exhausting because I couldn't help wondering why on earth some of my ideas weren't already happening? Super-simple stuff that would make huge differences (see pages 247–250) – which I guess is the sign of a solid idea. But one idea stuck out for me above all others. In response to the question, 'How could we encourage better support provision within all universities?', the answer I came up with was to make them compete.

We've all seen it – at every university open-day prospective students are bombarded by signs saying things like: 'Top 10 university for student satisfaction', 'Placed top five in employability leagues', or even, 'Ranked fourth of all universities beginning with the letter B'. Every year the marketing departments anxiously wait to see where they're ranked, scouring the plethora of random lists to find one they can show off about. The league tables found in *The Times Higher Education*, the *Guardian* and *Discover Uni* are the holy grail for university marketing departments. They are based upon the results of each year's National Student Survey. However, if you look at what they rank the universities on, you'll quickly discover that at no point do they thoroughly investigate mental health support. You can find out which university is ranked best for course satisfaction or teacher satisfaction; you can compare staff-to-student ratios, male-to-female ratios, and even annual spend per student ratios. But mental health support? Nope.

This strikes me as very odd. If you can evaluate how good an institution is at academic support, how can you fail to also evaluate how good it is at non-academic support? Some universities are introducing fantastic initiatives to support student wellbeing. Initiatives such as round-the-clock access to crisis support, fast and effective access to counselling, technology-based solutions to enable quick and effective contact. Meanwhile, other universities are prioritising none of those things. Instead they're trying to cover up student suicides to protect their reputation. It's screamingly obvious to me that we need to evaluate which universities are doing well at this and which aren't, right? Now that I've flagged it, aren't you curious to know?

I sure as hell was, so, very much in the spirit of September 2018, in January 2021 I started a petition to 'Include mental health support in university league tables'. In the description I wrote:

> This petition may not seem it, but the result of its success could be transformational. It would mean that in order for a university to be recognised as one of the best in the country, not only would it have to provide some of the best teaching and academic support, but importantly, it must also provide some of the best mental health support. The success of this petition would create a landslide cultural change – away from mental health support being viewed as simply a box-ticking exercise, but instead as an area to upscale in, to innovate in, and to excel in.

I genuinely believed – and still believe – that if we really want to change how these institutions address mental health support in the future, we must first know how well they're doing now – and make that knowledge public. Mental health support league tables will force institutions to take it seriously, giving them a financial and business incentive to innovate in the area. It's a sad fact that clearly students taking their own lives isn't incentive enough, but there we are. It wasn't long ago that we were locked in uni halls being tossed rotten food like caged animals. And if you think that's a shocking thing to say then you've proven my point: it *is* shocking and frankly inexcusable.

The petition quickly gained signatures, soon reaching 30,000 in May 2021, from students, parents and even university staff. A lecturer told me how annoyed he was at his department, piling on pressure and expecting students to cope without ever acknowledging that they might not be able to do so. The petition led to interviews with *The Times Higher Education*, the *Guardian*, The National Student Survey and The Office For Students. All of them said they'd look into it. *Eye roll*. And yes, it's still a work in progress – but the National Student Survey has launched a review of the survey questions, so hopefully, considering how important this topic is for so many students, we will see some changes soon.

A NEW DEATH, A NEW RAGE, A NEW VIDEO

In May 2021, a post was shared on social media about a student missing in Bristol. I have a large student following in the Bristol area so I shared it too. However, not long afterwards, I received a message request on Instagram with a link to a news story: the body of the student, whose name was Olisa Odukwe, had been found. He'd taken his own life. Fuck.

I propped my phone against a chair and pressed record, delivering my thoughts in a new video entitled: 'How many more times do I have to record this message?' (I won't include the transcript here, but you can find the video on my Instagram page.) After I posted it, I received messages from many of Olisa's friends in support and gained a lot of new names on the league table petition. I've actually been lucky enough to meet a few of both Olisa's and Finn's friends now and learn more about both of them. They sounded like wonderful guys and I wish I could have met them.

MY INVESTIGATION INTO HOW UNIVERSITIES RECORD STUDENT SUICIDES

'[The University] takes the prevention of suicide seriously.'
'The University is obviously very concerned to help students who may be facing a crisis.'
'The University's Student Services are very much alert to suicide prevention.'

In September 2021, I submitted a freedom of information (FOI) request to 121 UK universities, asking: *How many of your students have died by suicide in the last six years?* To clarify: it is a legal requirement for any public institution to respond to an FOI request within 20 working days (even if that response is just to say they need more time). Seven universities did not respond at all to my FOI, so are in breach of the Freedom of Information Act.

Of the 114 that did respond, you would assume that those claiming to 'take the prevention of suicide seriously', that are 'very concerned to help students' and that boast services 'very much alert to suicide prevention' would be able to answer this question with ease. It turns out, however, that the majority of them have no idea:

'The University does not hold this information as it does not record the cause of death.'

'Whilst we are always profoundly saddened to hear of anyone choosing to take their own life, we do not maintain a dataset tracking the number of people that do so.'

'The University of Exeter does not record the cause of a student's death as this is not a data item that Universities are required to report on statutorily, nor is it required as a business need to enable teaching and learning activities.'

Hold on, what did that last one just say?! That they don't record the cause of death of their students because they are not legally required to do so and there isn't a business need? What?!

A staggering 59 per cent of the universities that responded did not know how many of their students had died by suicide. I feel as though I hardly need to explain what the problem is here, but I can feel my blood starting to boil while I'm typing this, so please indulge me as I unpick this inexcusable and repulsive discovery.

First, you may be wondering if it's even possible for universities to find out this information – maybe it's a complicated process beset by legal hoops to jump through? Indeed, that was the impression I got from the many responses that went along the lines of: 'We don't know because "cause of death" is the coroner's decision, made at an inquest, and the university isn't necessarily notified of the result.' (An inquest is an inquiry into the circumstances of a death to determine how, when and where a person has died. It is based upon the findings of an investigation by an independent judicial officer called a coroner.)

On the face of it, this seems like a reasonable explanation. However, an inquest's verdict is publicly available information. To understand how easy (or difficult) it might be for a university to find out how one of their students died, I myself requested the verdict of my brother's inquest and timed myself to see how complicated the process was. It took me 52 seconds – and I received the response the next day.

Armed with this knowledge, I arranged an interview with a spokesperson from one of the universities that informed me they didn't record cause of death. That they didn't was news to the person I spoke to – he'd assumed they did. Clearly flustered, he said: 'I can kind of understand, I suppose, from a sense that we might not always be informed of that ... but I guess if it's gone to [the] coroner's we *would* have the ability to find that out.' Yes. You would.

Which led me to wonder why they don't? Fifty-nine per cent of the universities that responded were unwilling to spend *less than a minute* finding out why one of their students died. I think that is fucking unreal. This revelation brings up issues regarding both integrity and legality: why don't they record this data? I can only surmise it's because:

- they don't think they *have* to (no one is holding them to account);
- they've never considered it;
- they don't care.

For a long time, the guilt I experienced after Sam's death made me question whether I'd loved him enough. I hated myself because I interpreted previous thoughts and behaviour as proof I hadn't cared. I know how Sam died, I think about it every day. Sam's friends know how he died. My family knows how Sam died. Sam's school knows how he died. But strangers also know how he died – and much of that is tied up with the fact that it was suicide. Suicide is shocking and frightening, and prompts the kinds of questions that only arise after a sudden, unexpected and violent death. People want to know about it – and they remember it – because they *care*. Not because they have to know, but because they feel a need to know.

And here are all these universities saying, 'Oh sure, we care. This means a great deal to us. But find out about it? Nah, not our job. Not our responsibility. Not our remit.' Forgive me, but I can't make the two attitudes tally. How can you care about someone and then not find out how or why they died – especially when they were your responsibility at the time and that not only was their death possibly preventable, but educating yourself on the causes could possibly stop future deaths?

There is actually a law about caring, called 'Duty of Care'. Legally, an organisation has a responsibility to care for the people within it – this is applicable to schools, workplaces, hospitals, universities, and so forth. I'm now wondering whether the universities that don't record suicides are carrying out their legal duty of care? If a student dies by suicide, it's vital that a university tries to understand what happened. For example, by looking into the student's attendance, their engagement with their course, their living situation, support network, personal background, or any situations that might have contributed to the decision they made to take their own life. How can it do any of that if it doesn't even know how the student died? It isn't a stretch to call this negligence and to say that such negligence may be putting other students at risk of harm. As a comparison, if a student died by falling down some poorly maintained stairs on university property, you would imagine there would be an investigation, the stairs would be fixed and the university would likely apologise profusely and/or be sued for damages. But what if no one investigated? What if no one discovered that the stairs were dangerous? Could we confidently say that the students at that university were safe? Could we say that the university was fulfilling its duty of care?

Now imagine if over a hundred students fell down those same stairs in a 12-month period and all died. Are we really not going to ask any questions? Are we really not going to ask if there's anything that could have been done to prevent those deaths? Are we really going to feel satisfied when the university says, 'Yes, but look at all our staircases that students *haven't* fallen down!'

The previously mentioned University of Edinburgh investigation found that staff had failed to follow protocol and a student took her own life without being flagged to support services. As a result, the university was able to implement changes so that such a situation would be less likely to happen again. This aptly shows why knowledge, reaction and investigation are so important[6].

We find solutions to the mental health crisis not by focusing on what we already do, but by constantly looking for where we can do more. Not tracking suicide data suggests that universities are, what, simply not interested? I could tell you that universities only fund mental health services in order to be seen to do so – but I'd have no proof. However, I now have irrefutable proof that when a student dies, some universities don't attempt to find out how or why. The C.S. Lewis quote: 'Integrity is doing the right thing, even when no one is watching', is one of my favourites. Some universities need to have a long hard look in the mirror and ask themselves some uncomfortable questions about where their incentives lie.

From my FOI request, I discovered that in the past six academic years, 16 students from the University of Bristol have died by suicide. One of these was Natasha Abrahart, who took her own life while studying there in 2018[7]. During the initial inquest into her death[8], the Coroner ruled against considering whether the University complied with its legal duties in protecting Natasha. According to Gus Silverman, an associate solicitor representing the family, 'The University of Bristol has sought to dismiss concerns raised on behalf of Natasha's family by arguing that it is "Not subject to any statutory requirement to provide health services". The University objected to the family's request for the inquest to sit with a jury and submitted that there was no "legal or factual basis for intensive scrutiny of its actions".'

Her parents, Robert and Margaret Abrahart, have since launched a legal challenge[9] for a jury-led inquest into the university's role in her death, alleging neglect and disability discrimination (disability due to mental illness). The initial inquest heard how Natasha had disclosed to university staff that she had been self-harming, had previously attempted suicide and currently felt suicidal. At the time of writing, the new case is due to be heard in 2022.

Gus Silverman stated: 'There is an unfortunate and uncomfortable contrast between the arguments advanced by the University in this case and its other public pronouncements about wanting to learn lessons from the alarmingly high number of deaths amongst its students. It is to be hoped that the University will now reflect carefully on the meaningful changes it needs to make as a result of Natasha's death.'

Her father, Robert, said: 'The pain of losing Natasha is something that will never leave us. We know nothing will bring her back but we feel the University of Bristol should at least acknowledge what happened in the lead up to Natasha's death, show some remorse or regret, and apologise to her family. Until that happens how will the University prevent the same mistakes that we believe occurred from happening again?'

In a statement[10] the University of Bristol said: 'At Bristol we have reviewed everything we do and introduced a whole-institution approach to mental health and wellbeing with substantially strengthened support for our students in their accommodation, in academic schools and through central support services.'

As well as speaking to universities that don't record this data though, I also spoke to some that do and heard determination, empathy and compassion in their responses. One spokesperson replied: '[The university records this data] so it can be mindful of any memorial events (tree-plantings, for example) that may need to be marked, condolence letters or cards that should be sent out, or recording if the deceased student's degree certificate will be collected in their memory

WE FIND SOLUTIONS TO THE MENTAL HEALTH CRISIS NOT BY FOCUSING ON WHAT WE ALREADY DO, BUT BY CONSTANTLY LOOKING FOR WHERE WE CAN DO MORE.

by family or friends at a graduation ceremony . . . The information is also retained so that support can be made available for friends and colleagues of the deceased.'

Another spokesperson said she believes recording the data is 'really important' and explained how, if they identify a suicide, they 'make sure that we look after the rest of our cohort and find out where it's coming from and what's happening, so we can work harder to try and find out how we can support and make sure it doesn't happen again.'

In yet another, a mental health advisor told me: 'It's a privilege to do what we do.'

To the people who do care within universities, I say thank you. I want to acknowledge you. I also want to say: I'm sorry for your loss. It must be horrific seeing a student struggle and not be able to help, and I know what it's like to care and feel helpless. So, to the people who are trying to do good, please keep going and keep pushing for better. We need role models, and although genuine care shouldn't be something we should need to encourage, it seems that's the job we now have. I see you, I hear you and I'm with you.

MY PROPOSALS FOR CHANGE

I think one of the major problems we face with higher education institutions (other than the fact that a fair few of them can't be bothered to find out the cause of death of their students) is that the responsibility is put on students to reach out for support, when what we actually need is a proactive approach from the institution itself. Staff need to know how to identify at-risk students and how best to offer help. Symptoms of many mental illnesses are shame, isolationism, low self-esteem, exhaustion, lethargy, and so on. On top of that there's the stigma around admitting being unwell. Taking all of that on board, surely it's counterintuitive to expect people who don't *want* to seek support to actively do so? For some I'm sure it works fine, but that's exactly the problem – we've created a system that works for *some* people. Rather, we need a water-tight solution that accommodates everyone. In mid-2020, I was involved with a research study by Accenture that looked at the effect the pandemic had on the mental health of students in higher education. Twelve thousand students took part in the study and the results made for grim reading: 42 per cent of students said they'd thought about ending their own life; 73 per cent said they were frequently worried about not being good enough or doing well; and more than half (55 per cent) said that they felt lonely either every day or every week.

When asked about support offered by universities, the results were interesting. The most common university service used was in-house counselling, with 35 per cent saying they'd taken up the offer. However, of those who'd done it, 30 per cent said they didn't think it was effective. The most highly rated form of support was mentors or buddies – pairing new students with more experienced ones to offer personal guidance. Eighty per cent of people involved with those schemes reported finding them effective. However, only 14 per cent of people who had used university services reported being offered a buddy or mentor. Overnight support was the worst ranked service, with 69 per cent of people who had used it reporting it as ineffective.

Just under half of students, both with and without a mental health condition, reported that their university was 'doing well' when it came to supporting students with their mental health in general. And despite almost constant media coverage of the impact of the pandemic on young people's mental health, only just over a third felt that their university's response was effective. Importantly, students who said that their university did support good mental health in general (as well as during the pandemic) – and who also knew how to access help – were nearly three times *less* likely to say their mental health had declined since starting their course, and half as likely to be experiencing poor mental health at that moment.

At the conclusion of the study, I was asked to come up with suggestions as to what universities could do to improve the situation, and I'd like to share those with you now. These ideas are based upon conversations with an exhaustive list of people: professionals in mental health fields, policy experts, leaders in research, and university students and staff:

- **Improve service awareness.** Many people are confused as to what is available and how it can be accessed. This vagueness creates an unnecessary barrier for students.

Freshers week should be plastered with information about what to do if you're struggling – and then that messaging should continue throughout the year. Domino's pizza adverts are everywhere during that first week (you can't be a fresher in the UK and not get a free slice of pizza and a discount code on a leaflet) and yet I can't remember reading anything about what to do if I don't want to live any more alone in my room at 2 a.m.

- **Prioritise overnight support.** Enabling and publicising overnight crisis support must be an absolute priority for universities. SHOUT 85258, the national crisis text line, has a corporate partnership service enabling universities to outsource overnight support to it, for instance. Having a well-advertised, easily accessible and effective night support service is a literal life-saver.
- **Use attendance monitoring as a mental health flagging system.** Rather than responding to low attendance with a threatening, fear-invoking email, a university should use it as a golden ticket to identifying at-risk students. Anyone reporting as absent frequently should be considered vulnerable, contacted in a compassionate way and offered access to support.
- **Invoke a once-a-term compulsory student mental health survey.** Questions should be geared towards ascertaining whether a student is struggling and by how much; for example: 'In the past month, have you thought about suicide?' or 'Do you feel hopeless about the future?' They should then be contacted so that interventions can be put

in place if necessary. Those students who don't respond to the survey should also be contacted.

- **Investigate the mental health risk profile of students *before* they arrive and then proactively target interventions.** Understanding whether a new student has been under the care of a mental health service previously, or whether they would self-identify as struggling, will pre-emptively help to identify those who may need additional support.

- **Remove the cap on the amount of counselling sessions available for individual students.** At some universities students are eligible for a limited number of counselling sessions – and then that's it. So if they have six sessions in their first year, they can't have more regardless of changes in their personal situation.

- **Rigorously regulate support services.** Include a clear feedback system and record all suggestions or complaints, making sure they're followed up on.

- **Support services should reflect the needs of the students.** According to the Accenture research, the mentor/buddy support system was well thought of, and yet only a small minority of students report being involved in the scheme. Exploring rolling that out could be of value, but the onus must be on the universities to do the research. This is crucial in regards to ethnic minorities and/or the LGBTQ+ community, who may have different preferences and needs when it comes to support and what's most effective.

- **Every decision that affects students (i.e. in-person versus online teaching) must come under scrutiny for its impact on student mental health.** Contingency plans must then be implemented if necessary, should a decision be found to be detrimental. The university should proactively reach out to students affected and offer support.
- **All student-facing staff should be trained in mental health first aid.** Give staff the tools to teach compassionately and patiently – a far better long-term methodology than driving students to burnout.

There is much universities can do – and, even when they've done as much as they think they can, there will still be things to improve on. If this has struck a chord with you as a student, please exert pressure on your university to make these changes. There is no finishing line in the fight against suicide. It's about acknowledging that it's never going to be enough and can always be better.

TOP TIPS FOR STARTING HIGHER EDUCATION

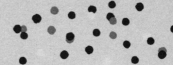

So you're on your way to higher education! Yes, it's daunting. No matter what anyone tells you – *everyone* feels nervous and anxious about it, and that's okay. Hell, it's totally normal. Here are some things that helped me when I started. Yep, I did drop out, so . . . I guess there's that . . . but a lot of these things are applicable in later life too; for example, when moving into shared housing, meeting new colleagues, learning how to strike a work/life balance and checking in with yourself.

If you're going to be living in student accommodation, bring a doorstop. Propping your door open will encourage people to stop and say hello. You'll also be able to overhear conversations and join in.

Keep a lighter on you. I don't smoke, but honestly I can't tell you the number of people I've met simply because they've asked for a light and I've had one.

Join societies. University is strange – you might not like anyone in your accommodation, you might not like anyone on your course, but that's okay! Those are people you've been randomly put with – you don't have to force yourself to get on. Joining societies that interest you is really important in finding people with similar interests, so check out all the clubs available. Things like: sports or quiz teams, radio and TV societies, the student newspaper, chess clubs and debate societies. Don't limit yourself to things you already

》》

know. The whole joy of uni is to try new things. (Apart from Magnums – yuck. If you know, you know.)

Try not to get too overwhelmed by work. I know, that's coming from a drop-out . . . But it can be super-daunting simply learning to adapt to a new way of life – so as long as you're keeping up, don't stress about it. Take your time and try to enjoy it. In my opinion, higher ed isn't only about getting a grade – it's about branching out on your own, testing yourself and meeting new people. However, if you are struggling with the work, have a conversation with your professor; at the end of the day you are paying them, so don't feel like you can't ask for flexibility or help. Who knows, your uni might have a buddy scheme through which they can connect you with a third-year student from your course. Also, lectures are actually pretty chill! There's this big hype around them and people make them seem so scary, but they're not at all.

Know yourself and give yourself the best chance of success. If you have a pre-existing mental health issue, make the university aware. If you suspect you may struggle anew, proactively investigate what support is available and make sure you're comfortable with what you'll need to do to access it. I do bash universities for their levels of support, but they will have some and if you engage with them early then the services can really help.

There's nothing wrong with not enjoying uni. You're not a 'failure' if you don't love it immediately or every second of the day. We've all had moments where we're like, 'Oh shit, what am I doing? I don't like this at all.' Admittedly for me, that period lasted a fairly long time, but almost everyone I know has experienced that at some point and got through it. It's important to recognise those feelings and act on them – can you join a club, speak to someone, change course (this is actually really common), invite friends or family to visit, or get a part-time job to meet people? Yes, you may end up leaving like I did. But you may not. Whatever you do though, don't squash the thoughts into the back of your head and pretend that you're coping for two and a half years, only to break down during your dissertation and drop out . . . Sorry, I went off on one there.

Honestly, it sounds cheesy but the best thing you can do at uni is just be yourself. It's a chance to find your herd, and being true to yourself will help you to find people who you genuinely fit in with.

TAKEAWAYS

- An average of 132 higher education students die from suicide each year in the UK. Many of them should have been offered support that is currently unavailable at lots of unis. We can all help to ensure that this changes by signing petitions, supporting the work of charities and individuals calling for change, and ensuring that we're equipped to have conversations with friends we are worried about.

- Fifty-nine per cent of universities that responded to my FOI request don't record the cause of death for students. This is dangerous and needs to change.

- Starting somewhere new is scary and that's okay. There are things you can do to better prepare and keep yourself happy and safe.

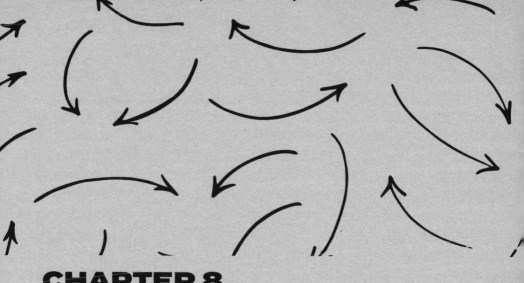

CHAPTER 8

A LETTER FROM THE FUTURE

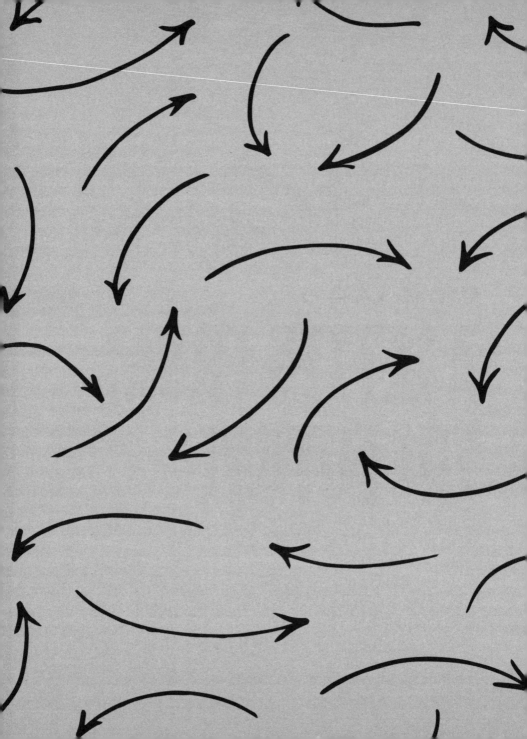

We need change. Change within ourselves and within our communities. I want this book to help progress both of those things. As I've said before, I really wish I'd never had to write it at all. I wish I'd never had to live this experience. I wish it hadn't happened to Sam. I wish suicide could have stayed one of those abstract things I only ever heard about on the news – something that happens to 'other' people. Like an earthquake. A remote disaster that prompts you to shake your head, say, 'Ahh, that's so sad,' but doesn't affect *you*. But it *was* Sam and it *is* me. And now that I am in this position, I want to use it to try to make sure that, if it can be prevented, no one else will ever have to be.

We've spoken about the need for education and mental health service reform – and people generally understand those aspects of this conversation. But there is still so much more to say. Here we are, in the last chapter, and I could go on and *on* about all of the things that are currently happening that shouldn't be or that aren't happening that should be. For a long time, it was claimed that the mental health crisis would be solved if everyone would just talk more – I hope this book has helped people to realise that while yes, that's definitely part of the solution, it's only one part. Many other essential parts aren't being talked about at all. For example, I bet you didn't know that mental health research in the UK has been described by the Mental Health Foundation as 'chronically underfunded' with only 5.5 per cent of the UK's research budget allocated to it – that's four times less than for cancer research.[1] The leading mental health research charity in the UK, MQ, published a report in 2019 showing how, across four years, an average of £124 million was allocated for mental health research compared to £612 million for cancer research. Twenty-five times more was spent on research per person with cancer (£208) than per person with a mental illness (£9). PTSD, ADHD, bipolar disorders, self-harm, eating disorders, suicide and OCD all receive less than 2 per cent of the total mental health research budget,[2] while research into mental health prevention (also described by MQ as 'significantly underfunded') receives only 3.9 per cent of the allocation. And, as if that wasn't all joyful enough, just over a quarter of the budget (26 per cent) is allocated towards children's and young people's mental health, despite 75 per cent of mental illnesses developing before the age of 18! How we can possibly justify this when suicide is the leading cause of death for adolescents aged 10 to 19 and the leading cause of death for all men aged 5 to 49?[3] No, I'm not saying we should stop investing in cancer research; I'm flagging up the disparity in research funding.

How can we possibly expect to make progress in treating, diagnosing and preventing mental illness if we don't prioritise research? It beggars belief that this isn't a conversation anyone in power is currently having. In MQ's own words:

'It's time to turn the hugely positive increase in attention on this issue into a public movement for action – driven by a recognition that research must play a central role in redefining the future of mental illness.'[4]

If you walk into a dark room, you'll bump into things. You can walk into the room a hundred times and, if you don't switch the bloody light on, you still won't be able to see anything. Those in charge are continuing to approach mental illness in the same way OVER AND OVER AGAIN. They don't change anything because they haven't done the work, and then they wonder why things are still crap. It's time we stopped tripping over ourselves in the dark and got ourselves a sodding torch. Or better yet, some strip lighting.

Shining a light on the issue is exactly what's been happening with cancer research. And it's saving lives. Cancer Research UK says that the survival rate of cancer has doubled in the past 40 years, from 24 per cent to 50 per cent.[5] That success has been achieved by extensive research into treatment, diagnosis and prevention – and we need to mirror that now with our approach to mental illness.

REFLECTIONS

When I was offered the chance to write a book, I thought long and hard about what I wanted to include and what I wanted it to be. I wanted it to be a catalyst for change, to uncover the truth about what young people have to navigate in dealing with their mental health, and I wanted to explain some of the horrors that I've witnessed – not for shock value, but as a wake-up call.

But the truth is, the more I've written, the more I've realised that, as much as this book was created to help others, it's actu-

THAT'S THE TRUTH ABOUT EMOTIONS: THEY NEED TO BE FELT. AND ONCE YOU FEEL THEM, THE BAD ONES LOSE THEIR POWER.

ally helped me a lot too. It's easy to avoid feelings – hell, I've been doing that for most of my life. And, looking back, I feel so hypocritical preaching about how important it is to talk about mental health and be open about your feelings, when I really wasn't being honest about mine. Not because I didn't want to be though, but because they hurt so much that I buried them deep within myself; so deep that sometimes I could almost convince myself that I'd forgotten they were there. Writing this book has forced those emotions to the surface, and, although it's not always been nice, I feel *so* much better for having done it.

That's the truth about emotions: they need to be felt. And once you feel them, the bad ones lose their power. It's not that they hurt less, it's that you gradually learn that you can cope with the feeling and that it will pass. Remember my balloon analogy? Well, over the past few years I've been blowing my balloon up and up and then up some more. I've been huffing all those crappy feelings into the balloon until it's come *very* close to popping. I think it's been stretched to capacity for a considerable amount of time (say, oh . . . since about 2018). But writing this book and being able to reveal so much to you, the reader (hello!), has expelled a huge amount of air from my balloon, and with that has come an extraordinary sense of relief.

Funnily enough, I really didn't expect this book to help *me*. I didn't expect to get so deep and so honest, but I'm really pleased that I have. It's kind of like an official record of my grief process. And once I realised that was the route this story had taken, I started to wonder how different things might have been had someone handed me this book while I was sitting under that tree the day after Sam died. Would reading about my journey through grief have helped 17-year-old me who had no idea what was to come? I hope so. I think so. But, bearing in mind that this version of me was sitting under a tree feeling like absolute shite and definitely didn't have time to read an entire book before heading off to school to pretend everything's normal, I thought maybe I'd summarise what I want to say to him in a letter instead. What key things would I want to tell myself if I could go back to that moment? Probably something like this:

Dear 17-year-old Ben,

Right now you're sitting under a tree and it feels as though your whole world has shattered into a million tiny pieces. I know how you feel because, well, I'm you – weird I know. Just go along with it, okay?

Knowing how you feel at this very moment, I'm not sure what to say to make you feel better. I could tell you it gets easier, but that would be a bit of a lie as it doesn't for a long time. It's going to be *so* hard, and it'll get worse before it gets better, I'm afraid. First and foremost though, I want to say how proud I am of you for the way you handled last night. I often wonder how I would have coped afterwards had I not known CPR or had I frozen like I did that time with Dwayne the leopard – but you handled it so well. Genuinely, you did everything you could to help and you should be really proud of that. Over the next few weeks you're going to doubt how proud of yourself you should be. In fact, you're actually going to really start to hate yourself. You're going to develop a very strong sense of guilt and shame, and you're going to convince yourself that you didn't love Sam, that Sam didn't love you, and that everything was your fault.

You'll soon discover that many other families that have lost people in a similar way also experience those emotions. They blame themselves and beat themselves up over times in which they feel they behaved 'badly' or 'could have done something differently'. You'll eventually realise − although it'll take a long time and, to be honest, you're still working on it now − that it was NOT your fault. I'll say it again, even though I know you won't believe me right now:

IT WAS NOT YOUR FAULT.

Yes, collectively as a society we are letting people with mental health issues down, so technically every mental-illness-influenced suicide is *our* fault (the royal 'we'). But hear this: Sam *did* love you, and you absolutely loved him − so much − and you still do. Suicide is a horrific thing that really makes you question your bond with someone, but you'll learn that Sam didn't choose to die, he was killed by an illness that made it impossible for him to do anything else. Man, I wish I could make you understand that right now, but grief and trauma do funny things to you. I mean, it's not funny at all − it's shit − but one of the things it does is make you feel incredible guilt and shame. That's a totally normal reaction to loss though. Feeling those things doesn't, in any way, mean you caused his death. Stop making everything about you, yeah? Silly bugger.

Brace yourself, mate, because life is going to be really awful for a while. In fact, it'll get so bad at points that I can't even warn you about much of what's to come because I simply don't remember it. Your brain is going to block out those memories as a form of self-protection (which is cool – you'll find learning about how the body reacts to trauma *super*-interesting). But I want to reassure you that you do get through it. Sure, you're going to go back to school this afternoon (and scare the crap out of everyone), desperate to find a way back to normality, and then quickly return home thinking, 'WTF was I doing?', but that's okay. People will tell you over and over again how you 'need to process this so you don't have problems later down the line'. But seriously – ignore them. It's absolutely fine to run away from those emotions and pretend to be happy and normal for a bit. Grief is excruciating and exhausting and draining, so you're well within your rights to choose to hide from it when you don't have the energy or stamina to do anything else.

Having said that though, you will abuse this allowance a little. While it's okay to avoid the feelings temporarily, it's not okay to pretend they're not there at all. You'll spend the next few months laughing and smiling on the outside to convince everyone (including yourself) that you're doing okay. You'll fabricate an illusion that everything's just peachy and you'll get lost in it. You'll forget that, actually, there's a shit-ton of stuff you're pushing down that needs to come to the surface. And, boy, does that end up biting you in the arse. So, I'll tell you this even though I know you're going to ignore it: feelings *have* to be felt to be freed. Please don't be afraid of feeling them sometimes instead of playing whack-a-mole any time they raise their head. Even if you don't want anyone else to know you're not doing okay, try to be honest with yourself and recognise when you might be feeling a certain way. Just by acknowledging the feelings they'll become easier to deal with, because you'll start understanding *why* you're feeling that way – and you'll stop beating yourself up for it.

I know you're probably thinking, 'Urg, how pathetic – "recognise your feelings" – who are you?!' Well, I'm *you* and being told how to deal with emotions was probably the most transformative lesson I've ever had. Honestly, fuck maths. This is so much more important. (Also, on the subject of maths: I might as well tell you now, turns out you're not very good at it. Go figure, eh? A degree in Aerospace Engineering is not a good idea. You'll spend two and a half years confused by numbers and end up literally laughing out loud in an exam hall because you can't answer a single question in the paper. Good luck with that.)

I know you want to act tough. I know you want to Deal With This Like A Man. But for God's sake Ben, hugging people and feeling emotions won't make your balls drop off. Unfortunately, you've been fed this narrative that you can't ever appear to be unhappy or as if you're not coping, and that's bullshit. Utter bullshit. Society has told you that being a man means you have to be stoic and tough, but that will only make you feel like shit. Yes, I get that certain situations aren't right to be sad in. Going for a drink at the pub with a group of people you don't know that well, for instance, may not be the best place to bring up how terrible you feel. It's not about having to open up to people in certain situations, it's about creating situations where you can open up. There's a difference. A situation like ... going for a walk perhaps. Do with that information what you will.

You'll learn all of this the hard way because you'll make mistakes and those mistakes will cause you to suffer ... but they'll also teach you things that will change your life. The next few months will be unbelievably shit, but you'll get through them day by day, sometimes hour by hour, and hell, sometimes even just minute by long, weary minute. You'll feel lost, you'll feel confused, and you won't know what's going to happen. And the funny thing is – no one could have possibly ever guessed what actually does happen. Don't laugh, but you're soon going to be writing your first book. I know, right? And so far, it's going pretty well (how do you like them apples, primary school?). Here's the thing though – you feature quite heavily in it. I hope that's okay? Tough shit if not. You'll understand why it's necessary soon.

It's 2022 now and the last few years have been a total whirlwind. And surprisingly, there have actually been some real high points – many of them entirely unexpected (like codeine being fucking awesome, for example). Your life is going to change beyond recognition and beyond anything you ever dreamed of. You become less aerospace engineer and more self-employed university drop-out. Sorry, yes, I forgot to mention that. You do drop out of university. It's because of that whole being shit at maths thing. But don't feel bad, it's one of the best decisions you ever make. If you could potentially make that decision a little sooner though, that would be much appreciated, thanks. You'd save yourself *a lot* of time and money. And, while we're on the subject of uni, I'd like to add that you should make sure to drink lots of water, both during your nights out and also when you're hungover. Oh Ben, don't make the mistake I did and get admitted to hospital for a hangover, sucking on bits of chicken because your jaw is swollen shut after your salivary gland explodes due to dehydration. It's a long story,

IT'S NOT ABOUT HAVING TO OPEN UP TO PEOPLE IN CERTAIN SITUATIONS, IT'S ABOUT CREATING SITUATIONS WHERE YOU CAN OPEN UP.

but trust me – save yourself a three-day hospital stay and just drink some damn water, please. (Although having said that, you do miss a maths exam while you're in hospital, so silver linings ...)

Anyway, I digress.

Why and how are you writing a book, I'm sure you're wondering, and what on earth is it about? Well, you're going to learn so many unbelievable things in the next couple of years about mental health that it will prompt you to kick-start a movement. Several movements! For starters, Sam wasn't alone in feeling really down about life. You'll discover how lots of people at school are dealing with some truly terrible shit and, while that's nothing to celebrate, they'll soon feel safe and confident enough to tell you about it. You! The person who, right now, doesn't even really know what mental illness is! Can you imagine the journey you're going to go on to get to the stage where *strangers* are telling you about their mental health?

You'll soon realise that more people are affected by poor mental health than not. You'll also discover how common suicide is – like, genuinely the number of people you meet who have a story to tell will scare the crap out of you. One day, you'll be having a conversation with someone in a bar and the manager will overhear you, come over, and tell you how both his brother and his cousin took their own lives. As he tells that story, another man on a different table will walk over and tell you how *his* dad took his own life. Right now, reading this as 17-year-old Ben, you're probably thinking: 'NO, THANK YOU. Why would I ever want to be having those conversations? That sounds like A NIGHTMARE.' That just goes to prove how much is going to change because, first, you're going to *want* to have those conversations. You're going to think having them is really *positive*. Second, you're actually going to seek out those kinds of chats. And third, you're going to share your own story a lot – and be okay with that.

Those conversations are going to be the first step of a four-year journey deep-diving into mental health, suicide and the support available (or lack thereof) for both. But what will shock you more than anything is how people seem to simply accept that suicide happens and that's just life. *C'est la vie.* What a shame. Onwards and upwards. Just this morning, you'll read an upbeat article[6] about how it's such great news that the suicide rate didn't increase during the first lockdown of 2021. Hurray, there were only 121.3 suspected suicides per month! You'll wonder if you're the only person that thinks the fact that the suicide rate stayed the same isn't something to high-five about. Yes, you know that many people anticipated that the stresses associated with lockdown would play a role in increasing suicide numbers, but the fact they're so high at all is still appalling. As is the fact that, during the Covid-19 pandemic, the number of urgent referrals to the adult mental health service reached the highest level ever recorded.[7] (Oh yes, Covid-19. How do I explain that? Hmm ... Perhaps that's a subject for another letter in another book.)

It's the same with universities. Oh man, give me strength. The number of people representing universities who will insist their institution is doing a good job because the data says it has a lower suicide rate than within the general population. Congratu-fucking-lations! Have a pat on the back, pal. Of course, *fewer* suicides is a good thing! But it's certainly not a good-enough thing. People really need to start learning the difference. And that's just from the ones that DO know how many of their students have died by suicide because, yeah, turns out that most of them don't! The truth is, Ben, that our family is one of around *twenty thousand* that have lost a loved one to suicide in just four years. Think about that – everything your family is feeling right now, multiplied by twenty thousand. That is the grim picture you'll start painting through hours and hours of research, investigations, conversations and campaigning.

Yes, campaigning! In a few months' time, you're going to attend an event where you'll meet someone who'll interrupt you, mid-angry rant, to say: 'You can't change what's happened, but you can change what happens next.' You'll realise he's right – you have no control over what's gone before, but total control over how you react to it. You can sit around feeling sorry for yourself and hard done by for a while – which you will and which you're more than entitled to do – or you can see the bigger picture, get up, speak up, and get shit done. Which, I'm proud to say, you also do.

One of the things that fires you up the most is discovering that, for many people in power – those with the ability to change things and really help people – 'mental health' is merely a buzzword, a catchphrase, a conversation to be seen having as a box-ticking exercise that only serves to mask the real tragedy unfolding every day. You realise you can help to bring awareness to the truth of the UK's mental health crisis by flagging up how saying, 'it's so important to talk and raise awareness' is as useful as an inflatable dartboard unless you offer safe spaces in which to have those talks, and the right support to enable having them at all.

A LETTER FROM THE FUTURE

Millions of people every year are reaching out for help, but the help isn't there. Health and social care funding is stretched paper-thin with departments so under-resourced that vulnerable people are falling through the cracks. Yes, people know how important mental health is, but do they know how difficult it is to get support on the NHS? And, even then, do they realise it may not be the right support? Do they know how poor some people's quality of care is when they do receive help? The number of mental health beds has fallen by 25 per cent since 2010 but the demand has increased by 21 per cent.[8] In mid-2021, you're going to read an article about how a mentally ill man was told by an NHS hospital that they didn't have any beds free for him. He was discharged so walked straight out of the hospital to a train station, jumped in front of a train and died. You're going to hear a lot of stories like that from people who have both attempted suicide themselves, have sought help, or who love someone who has.

They're horror stories. Horror stories from a national health service. How fucked up is that? Look, no system of that size is going to be perfect, and for all the bad stuff going on, there's a lot of wonderful stuff happening as well. The NHS is a fantastic institution and so many people working within it are hugely dedicated and heroic. The problem you'll have will not be with the many people trying their absolute hardest to make things better and to help everyone they can with the limited resources at their disposal. It's not even just with the fact that the system is broken. It's with the politicians and change makers who deny there is a problem at all and who spend all their time papering over the cracks rather than facing up to the truth.

You're going to advocate that the UK's mental health service undergoes a thorough inquiry into how it delivers care and what the quality of that care is – and that those findings are acted upon. Some of the statistics and facts will sicken and overwhelm you. You'll feel incredibly frustrated with how people don't seem to understand (or care) that many suicides are preventable.

You're going to start believing that the world is growing more fractured and selfish rather than less. Advances in technology that were meant to bring people closer together and increase connections will instead seem to have the opposite effect, pushing people apart. You'll start wondering if more people are finding commonalities in what they hate, rather than in what they love, and the internet will seem like a breeding ground for fury and despair. You'll marvel at how 'good deeds' become suspect. Perhaps this is unsurprising with Covid having exacerbated the wealth gap, pushing billionaires to try to justify their obscene bank balances by making a big song and dance about charity donations just to get everyone off their backs. People seem more cynical – which you'll discover first-hand when the work you do is lauded as remarkable and award-worthy, despite it being an entirely necessary no-brainer to you. You'll strongly believe that not having personal experience of something doesn't give you an excuse not to feel as outraged as you would if you did.

You won't believe this right now, sitting under that tree sobbing into your knees, but you're much stronger than you think – and you have something to say. And hopefully, your speaking out will encourage other people to do the same; to also realise that their voice has the power to evoke change. Real meaningful change that can define the future for people who, right now, don't feel well enough to speak up themselves.

Be warned though – you're going to rile people up. Turns out some folks don't trust people who feel strongly about injustice. Guess what you're going to be called? A snowflake. Yep, you'll find it wholly ironic that the generation fighting for climate justice, better mental health provision, equal rights and antiracism is called 'weak' by people who know strength only in what they can achieve for themselves. But, you see, here's the thing about snowflakes: on their own they don't pose much threat, but when enough of them come together they form an avalanche and their power can shake the earth. If young woke people are snowflakes – in that we show up time and time again, coming together as an unstoppable driving force for change – I'll wear that label proudly.

Every single one of us has a responsibility to create change – we can all do more. We *must* all do more. It is far too easy to deflect responsibility, to leave it up to someone else, and to secretly think that the onus lies with those who are suffering. But it's not their problem. It's *ours*. All of us know someone affected by a mental health issue. Every. Single. One. Of. Us. And the sooner we can accept that we have a role to play in solving that problem, the sooner we can make progress.

Right now, Ben, your life is in pieces, but you build it back in such an incredible and unexpected way. The change you want to see probably won't materialise for a while, the societal systems and structures you're going to target move at a glacially slow rate. But, regardless, I want to make a promise to you, 17-year-old Ben: I promise that I'm going to continue to beat this drum. I'm going to continue to write emails, send letters, meticulously go through research and government papers, attend events and tell my story. I'll give people a glimpse into what suicide is really like, meet with leaders, and make recommendations on what I believe should change. I'll continue to apply pressure to create change – and I'll do it because I care and I simply cannot cope with having to meet another family that's lost someone to suicide who didn't get the help they needed. I'll do it because I know the pain of suicide is one of the most raw and most excruciating that can be experienced, and because no one should have to face the darkness of mental illness alone.

I'll do it because I can't live in a world that accepts us *not* doing it.

But in return for that promise to you, you must promise me something – that you'll remember that when lots of people tell you that it's not your place to do this work, they're wrong. You're going to question your position a lot. Question what you're doing, whether you're worthy enough to do it, what business it is of yours, and how dare you think you have a say. And yes, the truth is that you might not be able to create change – you might spend all your time fighting only to achieve sweet FA. And that might feel like a failure. But get over yourself and crack on – because many of the people who rely on those changes can't fight for themselves.

There is a Jewish saying you're going to come to love: 'And whoever saves a life, it is considered as if he saved an entire world.' Sometimes it can feel overwhelming trying to change laws and challenge governments. It'll make you feel insignificant and small. But affecting just one life will truly feel like changing the world.

A LETTER FROM THE FUTURE

Think of life like walking along a path on the shore of a vast lake. Most people are so focused on the path that they don't notice the shore next to them or even the lake. They stomp along, as quickly as they can, trying to reach the goals they've set for themselves. Yet others *do* notice. They take the time to step off the path and wander about a bit. See what's going on. Maybe they'll even pick up a pebble and skim it across the lake's surface, watching the ever expanding ripples slowly distort and change the entire lake. Small things matter. Small changes matter. Small intentions matter. Simply by trying to change the world, you already have.

Ben (from the future)

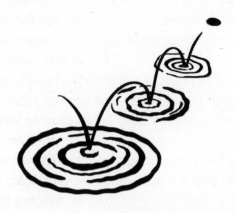

FINAL THOUGHTS

Well, there we have it – that's a wrap. I've written a book. What the fuck?! How totally random! I still can't quite believe it. Thank you so much for reading my story. It means a huge amount and I am deeply appreciative. And even if you skipped the whole book and are only reading this page, thank you as well. It's the thought that counts.

For those of you who did read the whole thing, I hope you found it helpful, informative, moving, relatable, funny in parts, and potentially even a little motivational (fingers crossed). I know things got pretty dark in places, but those places matter and talking about them is the only way of ensuring meaningful change. I hope you found some laughter among the sadness though – I always try to and, most of the time, it really helps.

I started campaigning with the goal of trying to save just one other person in Sam's position and one other family from going through what mine did. The way I see it, by reading this book you've helped me to get another step closer to achieving that. If you take one thing from what you've read – be it a self-help strategy, the impetus to learn CPR, the push to ask for or to offer support, or the desire to hold institutions and politicians to account – I'll consider it a job well done.

I'd like to ask that if you have been touched by anything you've read, please spread the word. Pass this book onto someone else who might gain from it, sign petitions, research the subject, support activists, ask a mate how they're doing, share your own story, be vulnerable, shout about mental health on social media, and organise your own version of Walk to Talk. Don't let mental health or suicide get swept under the rug and don't ever dismiss your feelings or assume that they aren't valid.

As much as there is a lot that needs to be done and a lot that needs to change, every conversation is progress. Whenever someone stands up, speaks out or seeks help, we get a bit closer to every person getting the support they need and deserve. We can do this. Together.

Above all though, I hope that reading this book reassures you that whatever your situation and however you feel, you are absolutely not alone.

Thank you for joining me on this journey.

All my best

Ben x

FINAL THOUGHTS

Ps I didn't want to end on a serious note so here's another top-quality shit joke:

Two wind turbines are standing in a field. One goes to the other, 'What sort of music are you into?'
The other says, 'Hmm. I'm a big metal fan.'

Yep, that's it, that's the end.

USEFUL WEBSITES/ RESOURCES/FURTHER READING

Shout 85258

www.giveusashout.org

Text SHOUT to 85258 anytime, 24/7, in the UK to receive free text-based support.

The Samaritans

www.samaritans.org

Call 116 123 for free anytime, 24/7, to speak to the Samaritans.

The Calm Zone

www.thecalmzone.net/2021/07/there-is-nothing-you-cant-talk-about/

A free helpline is available from 5 p.m. to midnight every day on 0800 58 58 58.

Papyrus

www.papyrus-uk.org/hopelineuk/

Call 0800 068 4141 or text 07860039967 for a free support line that's open from 9 a.m. to midnight every day of the year for young people that need support, as well as advice for those concerned that a young person may be suicidal.

Mind

www.mind.org.uk/information-support/a-z-mental-health/

Mind's A–Z of all things mental health.

Young Minds

www.youngminds.org.uk/young-person/blog/tips-for-talking -to-your-friends-about-your-mental-health/

Tips for talking to friends about mental health struggles.

Rethink Mental Illness

www.rethink.org/advice-and-information/carers-hub/

Information and support for carers of people suffering with a mental illness.

www.rethink.org/advice-and-information/about-mental-illness/learn -more-about-symptoms/worried-about-your-mental-health/

Information about mental illnesses and what you can do if you're concerned or need help. It also explains how getting support on the NHS works and how it's accessed.

NHS

www.nhs.uk/every-mind-matters
NHS Every Mind Matters campaign includes lots of information about self-care and strategies to support yourself or someone you care about.

www.nhs.uk/mental-health/feelings-symptoms-behaviours/feelings-and-symptoms/grief-bereavement-loss/
Information for people that have been bereaved.

BOOKS

Sisters and Brothers: Stories about the Death of a Sibling, by Julie Bentley and Simon Blake, ebook, 2020.
This Book Will Make You ... series by Dr Jessamy Hibberd and Jo Usmar, Quercus, 2017.
Book of Hope: 101 Voices on Overcoming Adversity, by Jonny Benjamin MBE and Britt Pflüger, Bluebird, 2021.
Reasons to Stay Alive, by Matt Haig, Canongate Books, 2015.

REFERENCES

Introduction

1. https://digital.nhs.uk/data-and-information/publications/statistical /adult-psychiatric-morbidity-survey/adult-psychiatric-morbidity -in-england-2007-results-of-a-household-survey.

2. Sadler, K., Vizard, T., Ford, T., Goodman, A., Goodman, R. and McManus, S. (2018), *Mental Health of Children and Young People in England, 2017: Trends and Characteristics*, Leeds: Health and Social Care Information Centre (NHS Digital, 2019).

3. https://assets.publishing.service.gov.uk/government/uploads /system/uploads/attachment_data/file/812539/Schools_Pupils_and _their_Characteristics_2019_Main_Text.pdf.

4. Saloni Dattani, Hannah Ritchie and Max Roser (2021), 'Mental Health', published online at OurWorldInData.org. Retrieved from https://ourworld indata.org/mental-health.

5. https://digital.nhs.uk/data-and-information/supplementary-infor mation/2020/waiting-times-for-children-and-young-peoples-mental -health-services-2019---2020-additional-statistics.

6. https://epi.org.uk/publications-and-research/access-to-child-and -adolescent-mental-health-services-in-2019/.

7. https://www.mind.org.uk/news-campaigns/news/mind-warns-of
-second-pandemic-as-it-reveals-more-people-in-mental-health-crisis
-than-ever-recorded-and-helpline-calls-soar/.

8. https://www.ons.gov.uk/peoplepopulationandcommunity/births
deathsandmarriages/deaths/bulletins/suicidesintheunitedkingdom
/2018registrations.

9. https://www.ons.gov.uk/peoplepopulationandcommunity/births
deathsandmarriages/deaths/bulletins/suicidesintheunitedkingdom
/2019registrations.

10. https://www.ons.gov.uk/peoplepopulationandcommunity/births
deathsandmarriages/deaths/bulletins/quarterlysuicidedeathregis
trationsinengland/2001to2019registrationsandquarter1jantomarto
quarter4octtodec2020provisionaldata.

11. https://www.nimh.nih.gov/health/publications/suicide-faq.

12. https://www.ons.gov.uk/peoplepopulationandcommunity/births
deathsandmarriages/deaths/bulletins/suicidesintheunitedkingdom
/2019registrations.

13. https://www.who.int/publications/i/item/9789240026643.

14. https://www.swlstg.nhs.uk/documents/related-documents/news-and
-events/reporting-guidelines/reporting-suicides/105-suicide-factsheet/file.

15. https://www.who.int/news-room/fact-sheets/detail/suicide.

16. https://thetab.com/uk/lancaster/2020/12/16/lancaster-fresher
-attempted-suicide-after-he-was-moved-to-empty-halls-building-22853.

Chapter 1

1. https://www.nice.org.uk/guidance/cg90/chapter/appendix-assessing
-depression-and-its-severity.

REFERENCES

2. https://www.thelancet.com/journals/lancet/article/PIIS0140-6736 (18)32279-7/fulltext.

3. https://www.mentalhealth.org.uk/statistics/mental-health-statistics -depression.

4. https://www.pnas.org/content/108/7/3017.

5. https://www.ncbi.nlm.nih.gov/pmc/articles/PMC60045/.

6. From *Robin Hood & Friends: A Musical* by Debbie Campbell.

7. https://www.accenture.com/_acnmedia/PDF-158/Accenture-Stu dent-Health-Research-Report.pdf#zoom=40.

Chapter 2

1. https://www.ons.gov.uk/peoplepopulationandcommunity/births deathsandmarriages/deaths/bulletins/suicidesintheunitedkingdom /2018registrations.

2. https://www.bhf.org.uk/how-you-can-help/how-to-save-a-life/how -to-do-cpr.

Chapter 3

1. Ministry of Defence, UK *Armed Forces Mental Health: Annual Summary & Trends Over Time, 2007/08–2018/19* (21 June 2019). Available from: assets.publishing.service.gov.uk.

2. https://www.health.com/condition/ptsd/ptsd-or-normal-post -traumatic-stress.

3. http://www.ptsdalliance.org.

4. https://bmjopen.bmj.com/content/6/1/e009948.

5. https://www.who.int/mental_health/suicide-prevention/exe _summary_english.pdf.

Chapter 4

1. https://www.samwestfoundation.org.
2. Office for National Statistics, Suicides in the UK: 2018 registrations (2019). Available from: ons.gov.uk.
3. https://www.mentalhealth.org.uk/a-to-z/m/men-and-mental -health.

Chapter 5

1. https://assets.publishing.service.gov.uk/government/uploads /system/uploads/attachment_data/file/664855/Transforming_children _and_young_people_s_mental_health_provision.pdf.
2. https://www.pshe-association.org.uk/sites/default/files/u26918 /ITE%20Report%20Feb%2019.pdf.
3. https://digital.nhs.uk/binaries/content/assets/website-assets /supplementary-information/supplementary-info-2020/10796_self _harm_suppressed.xlsx.
4. https://www.ncbi.nlm.nih.gov/pmc/articles/PMC1925038/.
5. Kessler, R.C., Berglund, P., Demler, O., Jin, R., Merikangas, K.R. and Walters, E.E., 'Lifetime Prevalence and Age-of-onset Distributions of DSM-IV Disorders in the National Comorbidity Survey Replication', *Archives of General Psychiatry* 62(6) (1 June 2005): 593. Available from archpsyc.jamanetwork.com; and Davies, S.C. (2014), *Annual Report of the Chief Medical Officer 2013 – Public Mental Health Priorities: Investing in the Evidence*. Available from: gov.uk.
6. https://www.ons.gov.uk/peoplepopulationandcommunity/births deathsandmarriages/deaths/bulletins/deathsregistrationsummary tables/2019.

REFERENCES

7. https://nhs-prod.global.ssl.fastly.net/binaries/content/assets/website-assets/supplementary-information/supplementary-info-2019/10774_anaphylactic-shock_suppressed.xlsx.

8. https://digital.nhs.uk/binaries/content/assets/website-assets/supplementary-information/supplementary-info-2020/10796_self_harm_suppressed.xlsx.

9. https://www.ons.gov.uk/peoplepopulationandcommunity/birthsdeathsandmarriages/deaths/datasets/suicidesintheunitedkingdomreferencetables.

10. https://www.ons.gov.uk/peoplepopulationandcommunity/birthsdeathsandmarriages/deaths/bulletins/deathsregistrationsummarytables/2019.

11. https://www.gov.uk/government/publications/relationships-education-relationships-and-sex-education-rse-and-health-education/physical-health-and-mental-wellbeing-primary-and-secondary.

12. https://www.gov.uk/government/publications/relationships-education-relationships-and-sex-education-rse-and-health-education/physical-health-and-mental-wellbeing-primary-and-secondary.

13. https://www.gov.uk/government/news/pm-launches-new-mission-to-put-prevention-at-the-top-of-the-mental-health-agenda.

Chapter 6

1. https://chiropractic-uk.co.uk/new-bca-research-shows-that-57-of-brits-are-moving-less-since-lockdown-began/.

2. https://www.workingwellglos.nhs.uk/wp-content/uploads/2019/01/Burnout-how-to-avoid-it.pdf.

3. https://asana.com/resources/anatomy-of-work.

4. https://www.theguardian.com/society/2021/sep/03/stress-test
-burnout-breaks-staff-recover-pandemic?CMP=Share_iOSApp
_Other.

Chapter 7

1. https://www.ons.gov.uk/peoplepopulationandcommunity/births
deathsandmarriages/deaths/adhocs/12336suicidesinfulltimestudents
aged18yearsandabovebysexregisteredinenglandandwalesbetween
2010and2019.
2. https://uclpimedia.com/online/if-id-have-died-i-dont-think-anyone
-would-have-noticed-an-investigation-into-the-harsh-reality-of-stu
dent-mental-health-at-ucl.
3. https://www.theguardian.com/education/2021/mar/16/edinburgh
-university-admits-failings-after-student-kills-herself-internal-review
-support-mental-health.
4. https://commonslibrary.parliament.uk/research-briefings/cbp
-7857/.
5. https://commonslibrary.parliament.uk/research-briefings/cbp
-9030/.
6. https://www.theguardian.com/education/2021/mar/16/edinburgh
-university-admits-failings-after-student-kills-herself-internal-review
-support-mental-health.
7. https://www.crowdjustice.com/case/natashainquest/
8. https://www.inquest.org.uk/natasha-abrahart-conclusion
9. https://www.irwinmitchell.com/news-and-insights/newsandme-
dia/2020/july/parents-of-university-of-bristol-student-bring-legal
-challenge-over-daughters-death

10. https://www.bristol.ac.uk/news/2019/may/natasha-abrahart-up-dated-statement-.html

Chapter 8

1. https://www.mentalhealth.org.uk/statistics/mental-health-statistics-research-costs.

2. https://www.mqmentalhealth.org/wp-content/uploads/UKMental HealthResearchFunding2014-2017digital.pdf.

3. https://www.ons.gov.uk/peoplepopulationandcommunity/births deathsandmarriages/deaths/bulletins/deathsregistrationsummary tables/2019

4. https://www.mqmentalhealth.org/wp-content/uploads/UKMental HealthResearchFunding2014-2017digital.pdf.

5. https://www.cancerresearchuk.org/health-professional/cancer -statistics/survival.

6. https://metro.co.uk/2021/04/20/uk-suicide-rates-have-not-increased -during-pandemic-14442610/.

7. https://www.theguardian.com/uk-news/2021/apr/09/extent-of -mental-health-crisis-in-england-at-terrifying-level.

8. https://www.theguardian.com/society/2021/jul/05/number-of-nhs -mental-health-beds-down-by-25-since-2010-analysis-shows.

ACKNOWLEDGEMENTS

Without the help of a number of wonderful people this book would not have been possible, so I'd like to take this opportunity to thank them.

Firstly to my editor, Jo Usmar. Thanks for helping me with the words – I think we can agree they're a pretty major part of this book. Thanks for putting up with and listening to the many hours of rambling, 'I don't have the slightest idea what's even going on anymore,' mid-breakdown WhatsApp voice notes. Thanks also for noticing that whaling is in fact very different to wailing, you helped me to avoid quite the scene. You've been a dream to work with on this – thank you.

Thanks also to the whole HarperCollins team who heard my story, felt my passion, and who have worked so hard to enable this book to happen. In particular: Holly Blood, Kelly Ellis, Julie MacBrayne, Tom Dunstan, Jessica Jackson, Ellie Game, Sarah Hammond, Sarah Burke and Ajda Vucicevic. Thank you so much for all your continued help and support. I know there will be many readers who will want to thank you too for allowing this book to exist – it has the power to save lives and that's only possible because of all of you.

I want to thank my whole management team at M&C Saatchi Social, but in particular Guy Warren-Thomas, who supported me throughout this process so patiently and continues to do so in all my work. You are such a gem and it's a pleasure being able to work with you. Thank you for all you've done for me, it genuinely means a huge amount.